Pediatric Ocular Surface Disease

Aisha Traish • Vivian Paraskevi Douglas
Editors

Pediatric Ocular Surface Disease

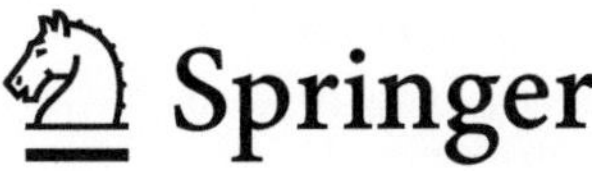 Springer

Editors
Aisha Traish (iD)
Department of Ophthalmology
Massachusetts Eye and Ear/Harvard
Medical School
Boston, MA, USA

Vivian Paraskevi Douglas (iD)
Department of Ophthalmology
Massachusetts Eye and Ear/Harvard
Medical School
Boston, MA, USA

ISBN 978-3-031-30564-1   ISBN 978-3-031-30562-7   (eBook)
https://doi.org/10.1007/978-3-031-30562-7

This Springer imprint is published by the registered company Springer Nature Switzerland AG
The registered company address is: Gewerbestrasse 11, 6330 Cham, Switzerland

Preface

Our vision for this book is to enlighten readers who wish to become more versatile with the diseases of the ocular surface in children. These diseases in children can be difficult to diagnose, and the ocular surface literature in this age group is limited. The consequences of misdiagnosis and delayed diagnosis can have a profound impact on their quality of life and ultimate visual potential, especially in cases of visually significant scarring and amblyopia.

Unlike adults, children are often unable to express their symptoms as clearly and examinations may be challenging. Thus, it is critical to develop a more complete differential in order to more accurately diagnose their disease. We did not set out to exhaustively cover every disease possible; instead, we chose to focus on some diseases that are common and would benefit from an updated detailed review such as vernal keratoconjunctivitis and those less common but potentially harmful if not recognized, including Stevens-Johnson syndrome and neurotrophic keratopathy. We are immensely grateful for the thoughtful and rich chapters that our expert authors have contributed.

In addition to the disease content, we wanted to share the practical surgical techniques and scleral lens experience of our colleagues and hope that these will be valuable for those who seek treatment options in this young population. We are optimistic that continuing to share the successful approaches of seasoned and dedicated providers will enable children to access the best therapeutic approaches and ultimately reduce ocular morbidity during childhood and for the rest of their lives.

Boston, MA, USA
Boston, MA, USA

Aisha Traish
Vivian Paraskevi Douglas

Acknowledgments

My foray into pediatric cornea came with my first serendipitous academic position at the University of Illinois, Chicago, in 2010, when Dr. Dimitri Azar encouraged me to consider this subspecialty niche. As a newly graduated fellow inspired by my extraordinary cornea mentors Dr. Claes Dohlman and Dr. James Chodosh, I decided to take the leap. I immediately fell in love with the unique presentations of corneal diseases in this population and the incredible resilience of these children with invaluable mentorship from Dr. Joel Sugar, Dr. Elmer Tu, Dr. Soledad Cortina, and Dr. Ali Djalilian and collaboration with Dr. Iris Kassem.

After returning to my training institution as faculty in 2018, I sought mentorship from Dr. Reza Dana and thus began the process of this book. I am truly grateful for every mentor as I have grown as a clinician from all the unique perspectives that they have shared.

Most recently, I have had the privilege of caring for patients at Boston Children's Hospital and Mass Eye and Ear and have been grateful to collaborate with Dr. Haji Saeed and Dr. Thomas Dohlman in the pediatric cornea service with unwavering support from Dr. David Hunter.

However, this project would not have been possible without the incredible collaboration of Vivian Paraskevi Douglas. Her dedication to research in the field of ophthalmology is admirable, and her meticulous attention to detail and critical analysis in our editing of these chapters truly benefit the reader.

Aisha Traish, MD

I would like to thank my mother Sofia, my father Andreas, and my brother Konstantinos for their love and continued support. I would also like to thank my mentors for their guidance. This book would not have been possible without the inspirational guidance of Dr. Aisha Traish and the valuable contribution of all the authors who magnanimously shared their knowledge and expertise.

Vivian Paraskevi Douglas, MD, DVM, MBA, MSc

Contents

Contributors

Manokamna Agarwal Department of Ophthalmology and Vision Sciences, Hospital for Sick Children, Toronto, ON, Canada

Asim Ali Department of Ophthalmology and Vision Sciences, Hospital for Sick Children, Toronto, ON, Canada

Department of Ophthalmology and Vision Sciences, University of Toronto, Toronto, ON, Canada

Daniel Brocks BostonSight, Needham, MA, USA

Karen G. Carrasquillo BostonSight, Needham, MA, USA

Angela Y. Chang Department of Ophthalmology, Scheie Eye Institute, University of Pennsylvania, Philadelphia, PA, USA

Piseth Dalin Chea Cornea and External Diseases, Jules Stein Eye Institute, University of California, Los Angeles, CA, USA

Calmette Hospital, Phnom Penh, Cambodia

Nathan Lollins Cheung Department of Pediatric Ophthalmology, Duke University, Durham, NC, USA

Jenny C. Dohlman Department of Ophthalmology, Boston Children's Hospital, Harvard Medical School, Boston, MA, USA

Thomas H. Dohlman Cornea Service, Massachusetts Eye and Ear, Department of Ophthalmology, Harvard Medical School, Boston, MA, USA

Konstantinos A. A. Douglas Department of Ophthalmology, Massachusetts Eye and Ear/Harvard Medical School, Boston, MA, USA

Vivian Paraskevi Douglas Department of Ophthalmology, Massachusetts Eye and Ear/Harvard Medical School, Boston, MA, USA

Abdelrahman M. Elhusseiny Department of Ophthalmology, Harvey and Bernice Jones Eye Institute, University of Arkansas for Medical Sciences, Little Rock, AR, USA

Department of Ophthalmology, Boston Children's Hospital, Harvard Medical School, Boston, MA, USA

Pediatric Ophthalmology, Cornea and External Diseases, Jules Stein Eye Institute, University of California, Los Angeles, CA, USA

Simon S. M. Fung Department of Ophthalmology, University of California, Los Angeles, CA, USA

Pediatric Ophthalmology, Cornea and External Diseases, Jules Stein Eye Institute, University of California, Los Angeles, CA, USA

Catherine Liu Cornea Service, Massachusetts Eye and Ear, Department of Ophthalmology, Harvard Medical School, Boston, MA, USA

Kamiar Mireskandari Department of Ophthalmology and Vision Sciences, Hospital for Sick Children, Toronto, ON, Canada

Department of Ophthalmology and Vision Sciences, University of Toronto, Toronto, ON, Canada

Lakshman Mulpuri Department of Cornea and External Disease, Bascom Palmer Eye Institute, Miami, FL, USA

Christina Prescott Department of Ophthalmology, NYU Langone Health, Grossman School of Medicine, New York, NY, USA

Kellen Riccobono Cornea and Contact Lens Department, New England College of Optometry, Boston, MA, USA

Hajirah N. Saeed Department of Ophthalmology, Illinois Eye and Ear Infirmary, University of Illinois at Chicago, Chicago, IL, USA

Department of Ophthalmology, Loyola University Medical Center, Maywood, IL, USA

Department of Ophthalmology, Massachusetts Eye and Ear, Harvard Medical School, Boston, MA, USA

Leyla Yavuz Saricay Department of Ophthalmology, Boston Children's Hospital, Harvard Medical School, Boston, MA, USA

Emmanuel Angelo Sarmiento Division of Ophthalmology, Cook County Health, Chicago, IL, USA

Reem H. ElSheikh Department of Ophthalmology, Harvey and Bernice Jones Eye Institute, University of Arkansas for Medical Sciences, Little Rock, AR, USA

Department of Ophthalmology, Kasr Al-Ainy Hospitals, Cairo University, Cairo, Egypt

Anna M. Stagner Massachusetts Eye and Ear Infirmary, Department of Ophthalmology, Harvard Medical School, Boston, MA, USA

Lisa Thompson Division of Ophthalmology, Cook County Health, Chicago, IL, USA

Danielle Trief Department of Ophthalmology, Edward S. Harkness Eye Institute, Columbia University Irving Medical Center, New York, NY, USA

Adanna Udeh Department of Ophthalmology, NYU Langone Health, Grossman School of Medicine, New York, NY, USA

Shudan Wang Cornea Service, Massachusetts Eye and Ear, Department of Ophthalmology, Harvard Medical School, Boston, MA, USA

Prashant Yadav Massachusetts Eye and Ear Infirmary, Department of Ophthalmology, Harvard Medical School, Boston, MA, USA

Dorian Zeidenweber Cornea and External Diseases, Jules Stein Eye Institute, University of California, Los Angeles, CA, USA

Chapter 1
Ocular Surface Anatomy and Physiology

Konstantinos A. A. Douglas and Vivian Paraskevi Douglas

Introduction

The ocular surface (OS) is a complex apparatus which plays an indispensable role in the maintenance of visual function. In 1978, Richard Thoft was the first to introduce the term "ocular surface" in an effort to delineate its anatomic limits where he included the eyelids, cornea, conjunctiva, and lacrimal glands [1]. In 2007, Gipson gave a more detailed description of what the "Ocular Surface System" term encompasses and defined it is as a system including *the surface and glandular epithelia of the cornea, conjunctiva, lacrimal gland, accessory lacrimal glands, and meibomian gland, and their apical (tears) and basal (connective tissue) matrices, the eyelashes with their associated glands of Moll and Zeis, those components of the eyelids responsible for the blink, and the nasolacrimal duct* [2]. In this chapter, we summarize the anatomy and physiology of all the components that constitute the ocular surface system and provide a number of protective barriers.

The Eyelids (Palpebrae)

The eyelids consist of an upper and lower eyelid which meet at the medial and lateral canthi, and their main functions are to provide mechanical protection to the eye from external factors and promote the distribution of tears over the ocular surface.

Structurally, the eyelids are divided into the anterior lamella which includes the skin and orbicularis oculi muscular layer and the posterior lamella which consists of the tarsal plate and palpebral conjunctiva.

K. A. A. Douglas · V. P. Douglas (✉)
Department of Ophthalmology, Massachusetts Eye and Ear/Harvard Medical School, Boston, MA, USA

© The Author(s), under exclusive license to Springer Nature Switzerland AG 2023
A. Traish, V. P. Douglas (eds.), *Pediatric Ocular Surface Disease*,
https://doi.org/10.1007/978-3-031-30562-7_1

The **skin** of the eyelid is the thinnest part of the entire body (less than 1 mm thick) due to the lack of subcutaneous tissue and the scant presence of connective tissue which is found between the eyelid and orbicularis oculi. Its unique anatomy allows for free and constant movements for opening and closing the eyelids.

The **orbicularis oculi** muscle is a striated protractor muscle of the eyelid that is innervated by the cranial nerve VII (facial nerve) and is divided into three distinct parts; the pretarsal, the preseptal, and the orbital parts. Forced closure of the eyelid results from the activation of its orbital portion, whereas the pretarsal and preseptal parts are responsible for the spontaneous blink. The mean spontaneous blinking rate in neonates as determined from digital videographic recordings is 3.6 (±0.3) blinks/min and the mean interblink time 21.6 (±2.8) seconds. The lowest blink rates are seen in children of 0–17 weeks of age (2 blinks/min) and increases to 5 blinks/min at age of 36–53 weeks [3]. In adults, the average spontaneous blink rate is estimated to be 12–20 blinks/min [4].

Retractors of the eyelid are classified as upper and lower eyelid retractors and assist in the eye closure. The upper retractors of the eye are the levator, Muller's and frontalis muscles while capsulopalpebral fascia and the inferior tarsal muscles belong to the lower eyelid retractors.

The tarsal plate (or tarsus) is found in the posterior lamella extending from the orbital septum to the eyelid margin and is composed of dense fibrous tissue of about 1 mm to 1.5 mm thickness. Its central vertical height in the upper eyelid is 8 mm to 12 mm and 3.5 mm to 4 mm in the lower eyelid [5]. The Meibomian glands are holocrine-secreting sebaceous glands embedded in the tarsal plate (~25 in the upper and 20 in the lower eyelid) whose primary function is to produce and secrete the lipid layer (also known as meibum) of the precorneal film which prevents the evaporation of the aqueous part of the tear film [5, 6].

The **palpebral conjunctiva** is the most posterior part of the eyelid and consists of the marginal, the subtarsal, and the orbital conjunctiva [7].

The arterial supply to the eyelids is provided by the supraorbital and lacrimal branches of the ophthalmic artery which is a branch of the internal carotid artery as well as from the angular and superficial temporal arteries which arise from the external carotid artery. Anastomoses within the two systems lead to the formation of arterial arcades along the upper and lower eyelids, namely the marginal and the peripheral arcades. The marginal arcades are located in the tarsal plate 2–4 mm from the lid margin. The peripheral arcades which are located anterior to the Muller's muscle are only present in the upper eyelid [6].

The lymphatic drainage of the lateral two thirds of the upper eyelid and the lateral one third of the lower eyelid drain into the preauricular lymph nodes and then to the deep cervical nodes while the medial one third of the upper and the medial two thirds of the lower eyelids drain into the submandibular nodes [6].

The sensory innervation of the eyelids arises from the trigeminal cranial nerve (CN V) and the ophthalmic (V1) and maxillary (V2) branches. The supraorbital nerve innervates the upper eyelid and the forehead skin except for the midline vertical strip which is innervated by the supratrochlear nerve which also supplies the superior portion of the medial canthus, part of the upper eyelid, and the conjunctiva.

The inferior part of the medial canthus, the skin of the lateral nose as well as part of the conjunctiva and the nasolacrimal sac are innervated by the infratrochlear nerve. The sensory innervation of the lower eyelid is provided by the infraorbital and the zygomaticofacial nerves. The motor innervation of the eyelids is supplied by cranial nerves including the oculomotor (CN III) and facial (CN VII) nerves and sympathetic fibers [6].

The Cornea

The human cornea is a horizontally ellipsoid, dome-shaped, avascular and transparent tissue measuring 11–12 mm at the horizontal plane and 9–11 mm vertically (adults) [8]. It is located centrally and surrounded by the adjacent corneoscleral limbus, the conjunctiva and its adnexa [9]. The cornea consists of the following layers: epithelium, Bowman's layer, stroma, Descemet's membrane, endothelium, and the newly described pre-Descemet's acellular layer (Dua's layer) (Fig.1.1) [8, 10].

Embryologically, the development of the cornea begins as early as the 22nd day of gestation. The corneal epithelium derives from the neural surface ectoderm, the stroma derives from the mesenchyme, and the endothelium from the neural crest [12].

The **epithelium** of cornea is a nonkeratinized stratified squamous epithelium and also the outermost layer of the cornea which is composed of 5–7 cell layers of various types of cells with unique function. More specifically, there are 2–3 layers of flattened squamous cells apically whose main role is the formation and maintenance of a stable tear film and prevention of invasion of large molecules into deeper layers. This is achieved due to the presence of multiple microvilli and microplicae and the expression of membrane-associated mucins MUC1 and MUC16 which produce the surface glycocalyx, a key component for the maintenance of hydrophilicity and integrity of the surface [9]. Subapically there are 2–3 layers of wing cells which

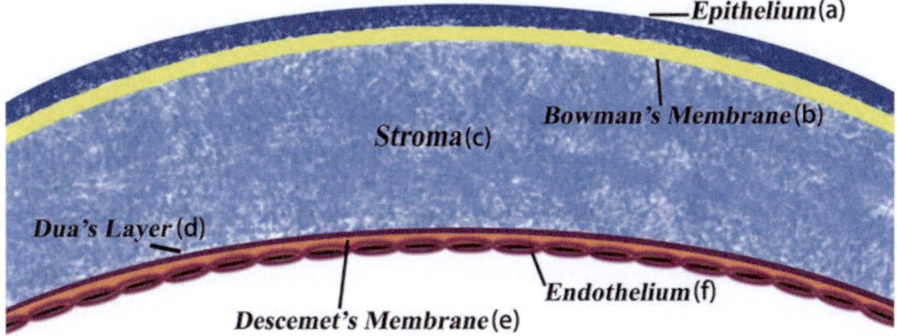

Fig. 1.1 Layers of the cornea (not to scale): (*a*) epithelium, (*b*) Bowman's layer, (*c*) stroma, (*d*) Dua's layer, (*e*) Descemet's membrane, (*f*) endothelium (Reproduced with permission by [11])

make up the intermediate layer of the corneal epithelium. These are cells at different stages of differentiation characterized by small size when compared to the squamous cells, darker cytoplasm, and poorly defined nuclei [13]. The innermost layer of the epithelium is the basal cell layer which consists of a single layer of cuboidal or columnar cells. The cells in this layer are the only mitotically active cells which eventually differentiate into wing and superficial squamous cells [8, 14]. Regeneration of the corneal epithelium occurs every 7–14 days. The central thickness of the epithelium is about 50 μm and gradually increases near the limbus (~1 mm). Apart from being an important mechanical barrier, the epithelium provides a smooth refractive surface along with the overlying tear film having a net refractive power of +43D (+48D of the anterior corneal surface and -5D of the posterior corneal surface) [11].

The **Bowman's layer** is a specialized, acellular, and non-regenerating layer located between the epithelium and the stroma and has a 8–14 μm thickness. It is mainly composed of randomly oriented collagen fibers type I, III, and V with unclear function. However, it is considered an important protective barrier for the subepithelial nerve plexus which is especially significant in cases of trauma [11].

The corneal **stroma** is a dense and specialized connective tissue layer which contributes about 90% of total corneal thickness. It is an immune privileged layer lacking both blood supply and lymphatic system [9]. It is composed of keratocytes and extracellular matrix which consists of type I, III, V and VI, XII, and XIV collagen fibers precisely arranged in lamellae parallel to the surface. The stroma is also rich in proteoglycans, namely keratan sulfate, dermatan, and chondroitin sulfate which contribute to its transparency [9]. The keratocytes are metabolically active cells which occupy almost 3% of the corneal stroma. Their density varies throughout the stroma but is highest anteriorly [9, 11].

The **pre-Descemet's or Dua's** layer is a distinct, strong, acellular layer of approximately 6–15 μm thickness located between the stroma and the Descemet's layer and is impervious to air [10]. This layer was first described in 2013 by Dua et al., and it consists of five to eight thin lamellae predominantly of type I collagen running in longitudinal, transverse, and oblique directions [10]. While the clinical implications of this layer have not been elucidated thus far, it is thought that it could serve as an anatomic landmark in posterior corneal surgeries and corneal transplantation [10].

The **Descemet's membrane (DM)** is a thick, acellular membrane which is secreted by the corneal endothelium. It is primarily made up of type IV, VII, VIII, XII collagen fibers, laminin, and fibronectin, and it is 8–10 μm thick [9, 11]. Embryologically, its development begins at about the eighth week of gestation where an anterior banded zone is formed while a posterior non-banded layer is synthesized and secreted by the endothelial cells across the adult lifespan [8, 11]. Descemet's membrane has a significant role in maintaining the corneal integrity, homeostasis, translucency, and overall corneal structure and curvature [15]. In addition, it has been demonstrated that within this layer, a bidirectional passage of nutrients, growth factors, and other molecules found in the aqueous humor occurs. This process highlights that Descemet's membrane serves as an important source of nutrients and a protective barrier [15]. When compared to the adult corneas, in infants type IV collagen (a1-a6 chains) as well as other components including nidogen-1, nidogen-2, laminin-411, laminin-511, perlecan, and netrin-4 are present in both parts of DM forming a railroad pattern, whereas in adult corneas, it is found only on its endothelial face [16]. Furthermore, type VIII collagen is mostly seen on the endothelial surface in the infant cornea and on the stromal aspect in the adult cornea [16]. In the study of Kabosova et al., it was noted that type XII collagen (long form) was positively stained on the endothelial DM part in infants and found in abundance in the adult corneal stroma [16]. Laminin-332, tenascin-C, and fibrillin-1 are seen only in the stromal face of infant DM. The findings from this study further support that the cornea undergoes a number of structural and functional changes from the infant period until adulthood.

The corneal **endothelium** is a mosaic monolayer of hexagonal cuboidal cells which is located at the posterior part of the cornea. Its thickness is approximately 5 μm with an average density of about 3000–4000 cells/mm^2 at birth and of 1500 and 3500 cells/mm^2 in the adults and in general is greater in paracentral and peripheral zones [11]. It has been estimated that each year the mitotic activity decreases approximately by 0.6% and this cell loss is compensated by an increase in the cell size variation (polymegathism) and shape (pleomorphism) [11]. Endothelium is a metabolically active layer whose primary function is to enable ion and fluid exchange between the stroma and the aqueous humor with the assistance of the Na(+)/K(+)-ATPase enzymes [9].

The cornea is an avascular yet highly innervated and sensitive tissue. A perilimbal plexus of blood vessels which is formed by anastomoses of the anterior ciliary artery (branch of the ophthalmic artery) and the facial branch of the external carotid artery provides metabolic support to the cornea with aqueous humor being the main source of nutrients [11, 17].

The innervation of the cornea is supported by the sensory nerves of the long ciliary nerve (branch of CN V1 nasociliary nerve) which run anteriorly in the suprachoroidal space and penetrate the sclera at a close distance to limbus. The perilimbal nerve plexus is formed from their branches which connect with the conjunctival nerves and further give rise to about 60–80 myelinated trunks that enter the cornea in the deep stroma. Thereafter and along the course of 1–2 mm, these nerves lose their myelin sheaths and three distinct nerve plexuses are formed: the stromal plexus which is located in the mid stroma, the subepithelial plexus which is found between the Bowman's layer and the anterior stroma, and the intraepithelial plexus whose fibers terminate at the wing cell layer [8, 11].

The Conjunctiva

The conjunctiva is a fine, translucent mucous membrane lining the inner surface of the eyelids and the anterior surface of the eye and extending from the limbus to the fornices [8]. A number of important functions are served by the conjunctiva

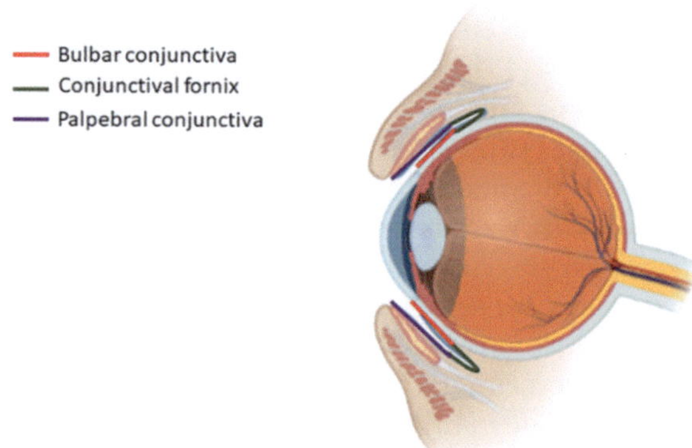

Fig. 1.2 Schematic diagram of the conjunctiva; bulbar (red), forniceal (green), palpebral (purple) (Reproduced with permission by [19])

including protection of the eye from foreign substances such as dust and microorganisms, maintenance of the moisture and lubrication of the ocular surface, support of smooth eye movements, and local immune surveillance [18]. The conjunctiva is divided into three parts: bulbar, forniceal, and palpebral conjunctiva (Fig. 1.2).

The bulbar conjunctiva is the finest and most translucent part of conjunctiva lining the eye. It is made of the limbal and the scleral conjunctivae, and it is loosely attached to the Tenon's capsule. Its epithelium is nonkeratinized stratified secretory epithelium overlying the basement membrane composed of predominantly type IV collagen fibers and the substantia propria which is a vascularized part with loose connective tissue [18]. In addition, a distinct feature of this layer is the presence of goblet cells that are apocrine secreting cells producing and secreting the mucin layer of the tear film upon parasympathetic activation [8, 18]. The bulbar conjunctiva receives its vascular supply from the anterior ciliary arteries and the peripheral tarsal arcades of the eyelids while the anterior ciliary veins and the peripheral conjunctival veins drain it before reaching the superior and inferior ophthalmic veins. With regard to the lymphatics, the nasal part drains to the submandibular nodes and the temporal part to the preauricular nodes. Sensory innervation derives from CN V1 [20].

The forniceal conjunctiva forms the intermediate part of the conjunctiva as a continuation of the skin. It is lined by a nonkeratinized stratified squamous epithelium consisting of a superficial layer with cylindrical cells, a middle layer of polyhedral cells, and a deep layer with cuboidal cells with scant presence of other types of cells throughout (goblet, melanocytes, dendritic cells) [18]. The vascular supply, venous, and lymphatic drainage are the same as those of the bulbar conjunctiva.

The palpebral conjunctiva covers the posterior part of the eyelid, and it is subdivided into the marginal, tarsal, and orbital conjunctiva. The marginal conjunctiva is 2 mm wide and extends from the eyelid margin to the tarsus. At this portion, the transition of epithelium from nonkeratinized stratified to cuboidal epithelium occurs. The tarsal conjunctiva is a fine, vascularized layer that is tightly attached to the tarsal plate. The orbital conjunctiva extends from tarsus to the fornix forming horizontal folds during eyelid movements [18]. Embedded in this layer are accessory lacrimal glands, glands of Wolfring, and the pseudoglands of Henle [18].

The palpebral conjunctiva has a dual blood supply with the main one arising from branches of the ophthalmic artery and additionally it is supported by branches of the facial artery. The post-tarsal veins of the eyelids, deep facial branches of the anterior facial vein, and the pterygoid plexus drain the deoxygenated blood. The eyelid lymphatics receive the lymphatic drainage of the palpebral conjunctiva and then drain into the submandibular and preauricular lymph nodes. Branches of CN V1 also innervate the palpebral conjunctiva, and studies have shown that vasoactive intestinal polypeptide (VIP)-containing nerve fibers innervate accessory lacrimal glands, goblet cells, and the glands of Moll [17].

The Sclera

The sclera is an opaque and elastic tissue forming the posterior 5/6 portion of the external eye. Its name is derived from the Greek word scleros = hard. It extends from the limbus (anteriorly) to the optic nerve (posteriorly) with its posterior part being the thickest (~1 mm) and the thinnest at the insertion of the extraocular muscles (~0.3 mm). It is further divided into three parts: the episclera, the sclera proper, and the lamina fusca [20]. The episclera is a thin and highly vascularized layer of connective tissue overlying the sclera proper and located under the Tenon's capsule. Its anterior portion is supplied by the anterior ciliary arteries and its posterior part by the posterior ciliary artery. The sclera proper (also substantia proper) is an avascular layer comprised by randomly arranged collagen fiber bundles of varying size giving the sclera its opaque appearance, strength, and resilience. The lamina fusca (also known as lamina suprachorioidea) is the innermost part of the sclera, and it is characterized by the presence of pigmented cells giving this layer a yellow-brown appearance. The anterior part of sclera is primarily innervated by the two long posterior ciliary nerves and its posterior part from the short posterior ciliary nerves [20].

The Tear Film

The tear film is a thin layer that consists of different ocular surface components originating from the lacrimal glands (main and accessory), the meibomian glands, eyelids as well as the corneal and conjunctival epithelium. The tear film serves many diverse and critical roles including mechanical, antimicrobial, and immunological protection of the ocular surface against environment factors, irritants, microorganisms, and foreign bodies. The tear film is composed of three layers: the outermost lipid, the aqueous, and the inner mucin layer (Fig. 1.3) [20]. As already

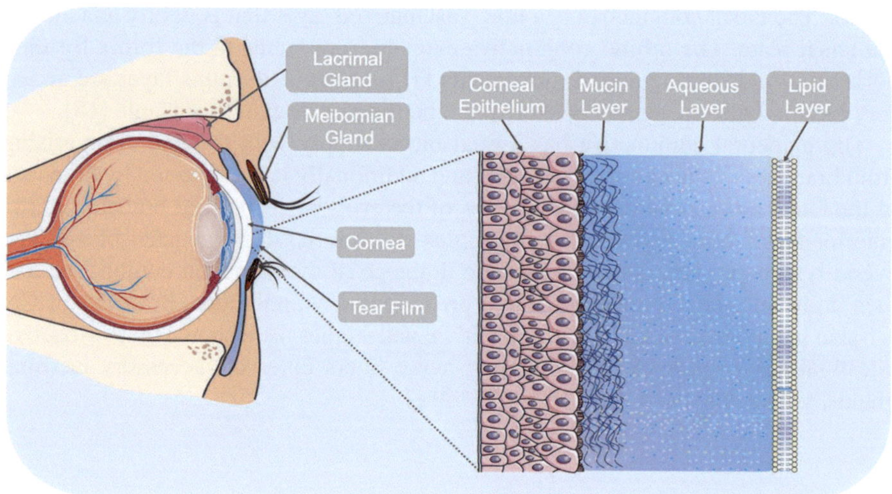

Fig. 1.3 The structure of the tear film. (Reproduced with permission by [24])

mentioned, the lipid layer is secreted by the meibomian glands of the upper and lower eyelids and plays an important role in maintaining a smooth refractive surface. Polar lipids (ceramides, cerebrosides, phospholipids) and non-polar lipids (cholesterol esters, free fatty acids, triglycerides) are mainly found in this layer [21]. The accessory lacrimal glands of Krause and Wolfring (non-reflex) secrete basally the aqueous component of the tear film while the main lacrimal glands are responsible for the reflex secretion of this layer. It contains water, electrolytes, glucose, proteins, oxygen, immunoglobulins, antioxidants, peptide growth factors, and other molecules [21]. The innermost layer, the mucin layer, is produced and secreted by the corneal and conjunctival epithelium which express transmembrane mucins (MUC 1, 2 and 4), the lacrimal glands (MUC 7), and the conjunctival goblet cells [20, 21].

The average goblet cell density in adults can range between 24 and 2226 cells/mm^2 with higher densities found in the superior and inferior bulbar conjunctiva and lower in the intrapalpebral exposed areas [22]. However, in the pediatric population, the densities are overall lower [4]. Dogru et al. demonstrated that the mean goblet cell density in premature babies is significantly reduced compared to term babies (393 ± 484 cells/mm^2 vs 739 ± 503 cells/mm^2, respectively) [23].

In the meta-analysis of Chidi-Egboka et al., it was shown that tear film osmolarity is higher in children than in adults with no sex and race predilection or clinical relevance [4]. However, it has also been observed that a number of ocular and systemic conditions can significantly affect the tear film osmolarity as, for example, diabetes [25]. In the study of Rohatgi et al., total, basal, and emotional tear secretions in full-term healthy neonates were evaluated and compared to those of healthy adults. It was demonstrated that at birth, 98% of infants had total tear secretion, 3.9% basal tear, and 2.9% emotional tear secretion comparable to those seen in adults and these infants reached the adult values within 12 h of birth [26].

Conclusion

In this chapter, a brief introduction of the basic anatomic and physiologic properties of this unique system is provided. Key differences between pediatric and adult populations are also included based on scientific evidence. Profound knowledge of the anatomy and physiology of the ocular surface is fundamental for better understanding the pathology of each disease as well as for timely diagnosis and effective management.

References

1. Thoft RA. Role of the ocular surface in destructive corneal disease. Trans Ophthalmol Soc U K (1962). 1978;98(3):339–42. PMID: 289214
2. Gipson IK. The ocular surface: the challenge to enable and protect vision. Invest Ophthalmol Vis Sci. 2007;48(10):4390.
3. Lawrenson JG, Birhah R, Murphy PJ. Tear-film lipid layer morphology and corneal sensation in the development of blinking in neonates and infants. J Anat. 2005;206(3):265–70.
4. Chidi-Egboka NC, Briggs NE, Jalbert I, Golebiowski B. The ocular surface in children: a review of current knowledge and meta-analysis of tear film stability and tear secretion in children. Ocul Surf. 2019;17(1):28–39.
5. Dutton JJ, Frueh BR. Eyelid anatomy and physiology with reference to blepharoptosis. Evaluation and Management of Blepharoptosis. 2011;13–26. https://doi.org/10.1007/978-0-387-92855-5_3.
6. Lin LK. Eyelid anatomy and function. Ocul Surf Dis. 2013:11–5.
7. Henriksson J, de Paiva C. Definition of the ocular surface. Ocul Surf. 2012:17–35. https://doi.org/10.1201/b13153-7/defi-nition-ocular-surface-louis-tong-wanwen-lan-andrea-petznick.
8. Sridhar MS. Anatomy of cornea and ocular surface. Indian J Ophthalmol. 2018;66(2):190.
9. Gonzalez-Andrades M, Argüeso P, Gipson I. Corneal anatomy. 2019;3–12. https://doi.org/10.1007/978-3-030-01304-2_1.
10. Dua HS, Faraj LA, Said DG, Gray T, Lowe J. Human corneal anatomy redefined: a novel pre-Descemet's layer (Dua's layer). Ophthalmology. 2013;120(9):1778–85.
11. Jacob S, Naveen P. Anatomy of the cornea. In: Jacob S, editor. Mastering endothelial keratoplasty: DSAEK, DMEK, E-DMEK, PDEK, air pump-assisted PDEK and others, vol. 1. New Delhi: Springer; 2016. p. 1–11. https://doi.org/10.1007/978-81-322-2818-9_1.
12. Lwigale PY. Corneal development: different cells from a common progenitor. Prog Mol Biol Transl Sci. 2015;134:43–59.
13. Sterenczak KA, Winter K, Sperlich K, Stahnke T, Linke S, Farrokhi S, et al. Morphological characterization of the human corneal epithelium by in vivo confocal laser scanning microscopy. Quant Imaging Med Surg. 2021;11(5):1737.
14. Beuerman RW, Pedroza L. Ultrastructure of the human cornea. Microsc Res Tech. 1996;33(4):320–35. https://doi.org/10.1002/(SICI)1097-0029(19960301)33:4<320::AID-JEMT3>3.0.CO.
15. de Oliveira RC, Wilson SE. Descemet's membrane development, structure, function and regeneration. Exp Eye Res. 2020;197:108090.
16. Kabosova A, Azar DT, Bannikov GA, Campbell KP, Durbeej M, Ghohestani RF, et al. Compositional differences between infant and adult human corneal basement membranes. Invest Ophthalmol Vis Sci. 2007;48(11):4989.
17. Krachmer JH, Mark J. Mannis, Holland E. J. Cornea. 1, China: Mosby/Elsevier; 2011.
18. Harvey T, Fernandez A, Patel R, Goldman D, Ciralsky J. Conjunctival anatomy and physiology. Ocul Surf Dis. 2013:23–7.

19. Hidalgo-Alvarez V, Dhowre HS, Kingston O, Sheridan C. Biofabrication of artificial stem cell niches in the anterior ocular segment. Bioengineering. 2021 Jun;8:135.
20. Tong L, Lan W, Petznick A. Definition of the ocular surface. Ocul Surf. 2012:1.
21. Foster J, Lee W. The tear film: anatomy, structure and function. Ocul Surf. 2013:17–21.
22. Doughty MJ. Goblet cells of the normal human bulbar conjunctiva and their assessment by impression cytology sampling. Ocul Surf. 2012;10(3):149–69.
23. Dogru M, Karakaya H, Baykara M, Özmen A, Koksal N, Goto E, et al. Tear function and ocular surface findings in premature and term babies. Ophthalmology. 2004;111(5):901–5.
24. Tashbayev B, Yazdani M, Arita R, Fineide F, Utheim T. Intense pulsed light treatment in meibomian gland dysfunction: a concise review. Ocul Surf. 2020;18(4):583–94.
25. Gunay M, Celik G, Yildiz E, Bardak H, Koc N, Kirmizibekmez H, et al. Ocular surface characteristics in diabetic children. Curr Eye Res. 2016;41(12):1526–31.
26. Rohatgi J, Gupta VP, Mittal S, Faridi MMA. Onset and pattern of tear secretions in full-term neonates. Orbit. 2005;24(4):231–8.

Chapter 2
Phlyctenular Disease, Ocular Rosacea, and the Role of the Eyelid Margin in Ocular Surface Diseases of Children

Danielle Trief and Angela Y. Chang

Introduction

Blepharokeratoconjunctivitis (BKC) is a chronic inflammatory pediatric ocular surface condition [1]. BKC is a clinical spectrum that encompasses staphylococcal phlyctenular disease, anterior and posterior blepharitis, meibomian gland dysfunction, recurrent chalazia, eyelid disease, and corneal neovascularization [1, 2].

BKC is a common condition in the pediatric population, with an incidence of approximately 15% [1, 3]. While some studies have found it to be more common in girls, other studies have found no differences in prevalence between genders [1, 2, 4, 5]. It presents around 4.1 years old, and because of its chronic nature, a specific corneal consultation is usually made later, at an average of 6.5 years old [1].

Eyelid margin disease, childhood rosacea, and phlyctentular disease are three interrelated conditions that can be manifestations of BKC. All three conditions are associated with staphylococcal hypersensitivity reactions. In children, these diseases often lead to more severe corneal manifestations than in adults and have the potential for permanent visual loss [1, 6]. The mainstay of treatment for these conditions is very similar and includes eyelid hygiene, antibacterial medications, and anti-inflammatory treatments [1, 2, 7].

D. Trief (✉)
Department of Ophthalmology, Edward S. Harkness Eye Institute, Columbia University Irving Medical Center, New York, NY, USA
e-mail: dft2102@cumc.columbia.edu

A. Y. Chang
Department of Ophthalmology, Scheie Eye Institute, University of Pennsylvania, Philadelphia, PA, USA
e-mail: angela.chang@pennmedicine.upenn.edu

A. Traish, V. P. Douglas (eds.), *Pediatric Ocular Surface Disease*,
https://doi.org/10.1007/978-3-031-30562-7_2

11

Eyelid Margin Disease

Presentation

Eyelid margin disease plays a key role in the pathogenesis of blepharokeratoconjunctivitis (BKC); and chronic inflammatory eyelid margin disease can lead to secondary involvement of the conjunctiva and cornea [3]. While eyelid margin disease is common in children, it is often underdiagnosed; one reason is its wide range of and often nonspecific clinical manifestations. Children may experience eye irritation, redness, epiphora, or photophobia, which can present as frequent eye rubbing. Chronic cases may present as recurrent episodes of conjunctivitis, chalazia, and corneal disease.

On examination, eyelid margin disease can present with eyelid inflammation, edema, thickening, hyperemia, injection, telangiectasia, eyelid crusting and scaling, anterior blepharitis, and posterior blepharitis, also known as meibomian gland disease (MGD) [3]. Figure 2.1 illustrates blepharitis and MGD. Blepharitis is inflammation of the eyelids. Anterior blepharitis is inflammation of the lash margin while posterior blepharitis involves the meibomian glands posterior to the lash margin. Anterior blepharitis, with presence of collarettes at the base of the eyelashes bases, can signify Demodex colonization. Demodex colonization has been associated with more severe eyelid margin inflammation and MGD [6]. In MGD, the meibomian glands may appear inflamed, inspissated, or clogged. One study found that in children with BKC, anterior blepharitis is more common than posterior blepharitis [3].

Even though blepharitis is common in children, BKC, or involvement of the cornea and conjunctiva is relatively rare [8]. However, untreated eyelid margin disease in children can also lead to corneal changes including punctate epithelial keratitis, marginal infiltrates, corneal ulceration, and corneal phlyctenules [3, 7]. Figure 2.2 shows a patient who developed a corneal infiltrate and scar in the setting of BKC. Corneal involvement in BKC often affects the inferior cornea, near the lid margin. More severe manifestations of BKC, such as corneal neovascularization,

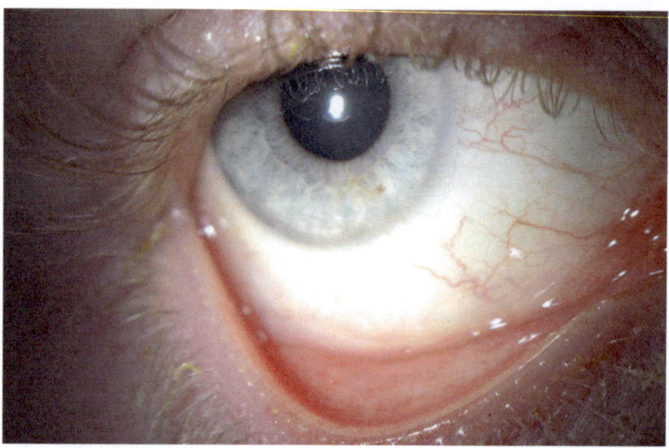

Fig. 2.1 Eyelid margin disease with meibomian gland disease and blepharitis. Eyelid crusting and scaling can be seen along the lash margins

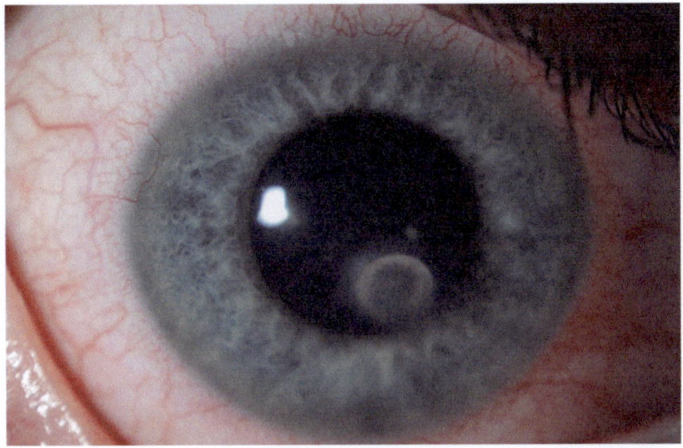

Fig. 2.2 Blepharokeratoconjunctivitis with subsequent development of corneal infiltrate and scar

corneal ulceration, and corneal scarring, are associated with children of Asian and Middle Eastern origin [7]. Rarely, chronic BKC can cause corneal perforation.

BKC is of particular concern in the pediatric population because of its potential to cause permanent visual loss. While the clinical manifestations of blepharitis and BKC may be similar among children and adults, children experience a more marked impact on their vision than would be expected [9]. Compared to adults, children are more likely to experience more severe corneal damage from BKC [6]. Children may also mount a greater immune response to colonized bacteria than adults, leading to corneal damage [9]. Sequalae including corneal neovascularization, corneal scarring, and ulceration can impair visual function through irregular astigmatism and refractive changes [3]. While BKC is typically bilateral, it can also be unilateral or asymmetric. For children, delayed treatment in severe cases of BKC can lead to amblyopia and permanent visual impairment due to chronic inflammation or induction of astigmatism [9].

Pathophysiology

In many cases, eyelid margin disease is associated with colonization of staphylococcal species, especially in more severe cases. The most implicated organism is *Staphylococcus aureus* and less commonly, *Staphylococcus epidermidis*. These antigens often lead to an immune-mediated keratitis and conjunctivitis that exists as part of the BKC clinical spectrum. Figure 2.3 shows staphylococcal marginal keratitis with the characteristic stromal infiltrates along the corneal limbus with an adjacent area of clearing. Blepharitis can cause a secondary immune-mediated reaction that leads to the clinical manifestations of BKC.

BKC in children differs from that in adults due to its more severe disease course with more frequent corneal involvement. The increase in severity in children could

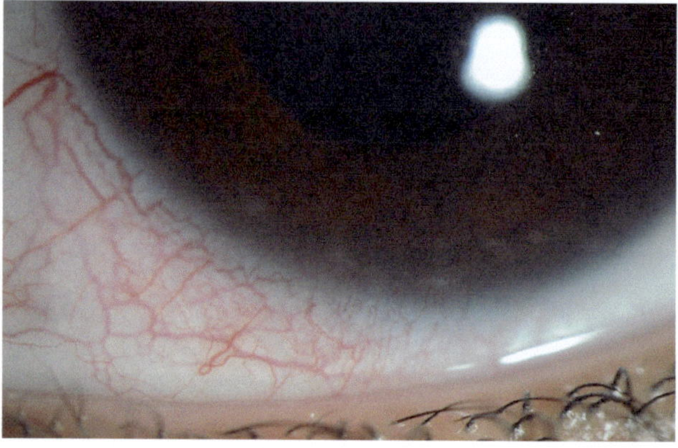

Fig. 2.3 Staphylococcal marginal keratitis. Stromal infiltrates are seen near the limbus of the cornea, with an adjacent area of clearing

be due to an immature and exaggerated response to bacterial antigens in the periocular area [9]. Another theory is that children may have immature corneal defenses against these bacteria [9]. The differences between disease course in children and adults could also be due to differences in their ocular flora. The conjunctival flora also differ between adults and children; *Propionibacterium* species are more commonly found in higher numbers in adults while *Streptococcus* species are more commonly found in children [10].

Treatment

While eyelid margin disease and BKC can be self-limited, especially early episodes, treatment is often required to control symptoms and prevent recurrence. Treatment relies on anti-inflammatory and antibacterial management as well as control of blepharitis.

For blepharitis, daily lid hygiene with warm compresses and an eyelid scrub is the mainstay of treatment. Lid hygiene with warm compresses removes debris on the eyelid margin and unclogs the meibomian glands by liquefying the thickened secretions, thus alleviating symptoms and improving the blepharitis. Often, it is necessary to continue the regimen of lid hygiene and warm compresses indefinitely to prevent disease recurrence. Artificial tears and other topical lubricants can be used to protect the ocular surface given tear film derangements. A challenge in treating BKC in children is compliance with a daily lid hygiene regimen as well as application of topical medications.

In more severe cases of blepharitis, systemic therapies may be indicated; doxycycline can be used to reduce the amount of inflammation at the eyelid margin and treat blepharitis. Of note, tetracyclines cannot be used in children under 8 years of age due to risk of tooth discoloration and negative impact on bone growth. In younger children, oral azithromycin or erythromycin can be used [8, 11, 12].

The underlying etiology for the BKC must be addressed as well, especially if it is infectious. Patients with active blepharitis can also undergo eyelid margin cultures or cultures of the conjunctival/corneal scrapings of the lesions. Children with BKC may have lid cultures that are positive for organisms including staphylococcal species, P. acnes, S. viridans, and chlamydia. Positive cultures can guide antibiotic selection for treatment. Antibiotics can include eyedrops during the day and ointment at the eyelid margin at night. More severe cases may require systemic antibiotics such as erythromycin [7]. Moreover, application of dilute hypochlorous acid sprays can also decrease the bacterial load.

Phlyctenular Disease

Pathophysiology

Phlyctenular keratoconjunctivitis (PKC) is inflammation of the cornea and conjunctiva caused by a hypersensitivity, delayed cell-mediated response to microbial antigens and is commonly seen in children [13–15].

Phlyctenular disease is characterized by phlyctenulosis, which is the development of hyperemic focal nodules that can occur on the cornea or conjunctiva. It typically presents in the first two decades of life and exhibits peaks in ages 3–4 years and 15 years [13]. Phlyctenular disease is more common in females [13, 15]. Phlyctenulosis also displays seasonal variation, with increased incidence in the spring between April and June [13].

Phlyctenular disease is most commonly associated with *Staphylococcus aureus* infection in developed countries [16]. *Staphylococcus aureus* is a common bacteria found in the eyelid margin, and sensitization to bacterial products, especially in the setting of chronic staphylococcal blepharitis, can lead to PKC. Positive conjunctival and lid cultures have been observed in phlyctenular disease, particularly for *Staphylococcus aureus*, *Staphylococcus epidermidis*, *and chlamydia* [4, 14]. Characteristically, children with PKC have heavy, confluent growth of *Staphylococcus aureus*.

In developing countries, phlyctenular disease is classically associated with mycobacterium tuberculosis (TB), as a hypersensitivity to tuberculoprotein [13, 15, 16]. PKC can arise in latent TB, active TB, and active TB undergoing multidrug therapy [16]. PKC can also occur as a result of a hypersensitivity reaction to the tuberculoprotein even in the absence of tuberculosis [13–15].

Of note, the type of antigen implicated in phlyctenular disease can lead to different manifestations; staphylococcal associated disease typically affects older individuals, causes less photophobia, and is less responsive to steroid treatment [16]. Additionally, recurrence and more severe disease (i.e., corneal phlyctens, multiple lesions, bilateral involvement) are associated with patients with tuberculosis [16]. Additionally, lesions on the cornea tend to be associated with diagnosis of TB [16]. Less frequently, chlamydia [4], candida albicans, parasitic [17] (i.e., hymenolepis nana, ascaris lumbricoides, ancylostoma duodenale), and viral infections [16] (herpes zoster) have also been implicated in phlyctenular disease [13, 18–20]. It should be noted that in studies of children with PKC, no associated infection could be identified with cultures in the majority of cases [14, 16].

Presentation

PKC often presents with foreign body sensation, photophobia, tearing, blepharo-spasm, irritation, and redness. Mild conjunctival discharge is often seen, but less frequently, mucopurulent conjunctivitis can also be observed [16]. Untreated or recurrent episodes of PKC can lead to corneal neovascularization and scarring. Corneal phlyctens are more likely to cause visual impairment. Rarely, PKC can lead to corneal thinning, perforation, secondary bacterial infection, and blindness [4, 5, 14, 21].

Phlyctenulosis is a nodular reaction in the conjunctiva or cornea [13]. PKC most commonly presents with limbal phlyctens: circumscribed subepithelial nodules arising at the corneal limbus [13, 15, 16]. Histopathological examination of the phlyctenular lesions reveals T lymphocytes, histiocytes, and plasma cells [22]. In the ulceration phase of the lesion, leukocytes are present [22].

As shown in Fig. 2.4, phlyctenules are most often observed at the limbus, though they can subsequently spread to the cornea or conjunctiva in one or both eyes [14]. Conjunctival phlyctenules are characterized as 1–3 mm pinkish-white nodules within an area of hyperemia [22]. Corneal and palpebral phlyctenules are more commonly observed in recurrent disease [16]. Corneal lesions can lead to visual impairment while conjunctival lesions are typically transient and asymptomatic [16]. Less commonly, linear (fascicular) corneal phlyctenules can be observed; phlyctens can migrate from the limbus toward the center of the cornea and lead to

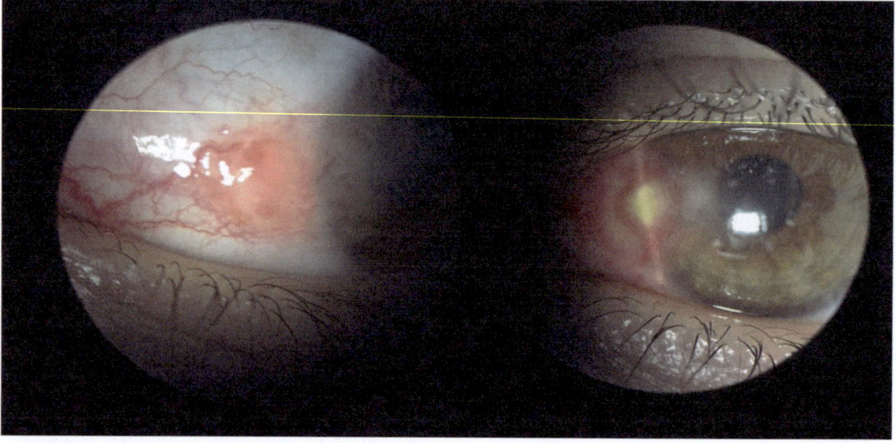

Fig. 2.4 Phlyctenule along the corneal limbus seen in phlyctenular keratoconjunctivitis. Courtesy of Dr. Jonathan Fay

neovascularization or pannus formation and subsequent scarring [4, 22]. Phlyctenules often last 2–3 weeks then resolve spontaneously. Toward the end of their course, phlycten sometimes develop into a microabscess that ulcerates and heals without scarring [14]. Differential diagnoses for PKC include pinguecula, nodular episcleritis, marginal corneal ulcer, and herpes simplex keratitis, vernal keratoconjunctivitis, and malignancy, especially if it is unilateral and refractory to treatment [22].

Treatment

Similar to the treatment discussed for eyelid margin disease, treatment of PKC relies primarily on decreasing the staphylococcal colonization, treating the blepharitis, and mitigating the local immune response [7].

The underlying etiology should be considered for every patient with phlyctenular disease. While topical and systemic treatment can lead to resolution of ocular symptoms, concomitant treatment of the underlying infection (i.e., TB, helminthiasis) is also crucial for preventing recurrence. Because of the strong association of phlyctenular disease and TB, every patient with phlyctenular disease should undergo TB testing with a PPD with anergy panel and a chest X-ray in the case of a positive PPD.

If infectious disease like TB is ruled out and PKC is thought to be inflammatory in nature, topical steroids are the pillar of treatment, especially during flares. Fluorometholone 1% has been found to be efficacious in treating PKC [14]. In cases of recurrent PKC, combination of topical steroid and antibiotics, such as dexamethasone 0.01% and tobramycin 0.3%, has been used [14]. Although topical steroids can be quite effective in treating PKC, care must be taken to prevent steroid dependence, especially because there is frequent recurrence of disease in these children. One study examining children with PKC experiencing steroid-dependent corneal inflammation found that cyclosporine 2% was efficacious for treatment of PKC [23]. Topical tacrolimus 0.03% ointment has also been used in treating severe, refractory PKC or as maintenance therapy in recurrent steroid-dependent cases [24, 25]. Tacrolimus is an immunosuppressive macrolide that suppresses T cell activation. Since PKC involves T cell-mediated hypersensitivity, tacrolimus has been used successfully as treatment in cases that have been refractory to other therapies [24, 25]. Tacrolimus does, however, carry a black box warning for a potential association with secondary lymphoproliferative disease in animals [24, 26].

While steroids can be effective for controlling symptoms, flares may occur when steroid treatment is stopped. Additionally, when the disease is associated with staphylococcal infection, steroid treatment may be less effective, especially if the inciting agent, the bacterial infection, is left untreated. Courses of oral tetracycline or erythromycin have also been found to produce long-lasting remission of PKC, especially in staphylococcal PKC or in children with steroid-induced complications [4, 5]. Another study showed that azithromycin 1.5% eye drops was also effective in treating PKC [27]. Adjuvant topical steroid therapy may be used to prevent recurrence. Patients with symptomatic photophobia or significant corneal involvement may also benefit from cycloplegic eye drops.

Childhood Rosacea

Presentation

Rosacea is a dermatologic condition that usually affects the face and can have ocular manifestations. The cutaneous manifestations include facial erythema, telangiectasias, flushing, papules, pustules, and sebaceous gland hypertrophy on the cheeks, chin, forehead, and nasolabial folds [28]. Figure 2.5 illustrates an example of ocular rosacea with telangiectasias seen at the eyelid margin. Rosacea can also have ophthalmic manifestations. Ocular rosacea in children is more commonly seen in girls and is often bilateral [28]. It can lead to nonspecific ocular symptoms with blurred vision, redness, burning, and itching, leading to underdiagnosis or misdiagnosis. Other types of ocular manifestations include blepharitis, MGD, conjunctivitis, recurrent chalazia, episcleritis, episcleritis, keratitis, corneal scarring, and BKC [29]. Ocular involvement of rosacea can occur in conjunction or independently of cutaneous rosacea. Approximately 58% of patients with rosacea have ocular manifestations [30]. Although rosacea most commonly affects adults, usually women, presenting at 30–50 years old, it can similarly manifest in children, especially in those with BKC [27, 29, 31].

Rosacea in children is thought to be part of the clinical spectrum for BKC. In children, the disease can manifest with the characteristic inflammatory cutaneous involvement on the face. However, it is often difficult to diagnose children with rosacea because of the lack of validated diagnostic criteria in children; the characteristic skin changes seen in adults may not be seen in children with rosacea, particularly before puberty [12]. Additionally, particularly in children, ocular symptoms can precede dermatologic manifestation. However, in children, ocular manifestations of rosacea are rare, especially before puberty [29].

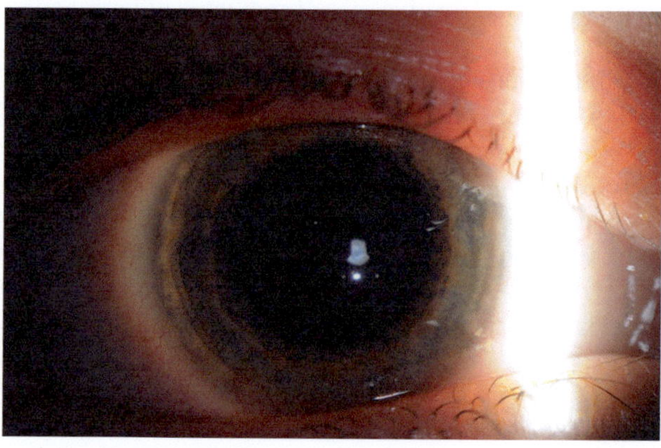

Fig. 2.5 Ocular rosacea with telangiectasias along eyelid margin with conjunctival injection and corneal neovascularization at the corneal limbus

Additionally, ocular-only manifestations of rosacea may be difficult to differentiate from other types of ocular surface disease that present similarly. Ocular rosacea should specifically be suspected if there are lid margin telangiectasias, meibomian gland dysfunction or blepharitis, and a long history of persistent ocular surface disease that has failed first-line treatments. In children with concomitant skin symptoms, the typical findings of facial flushing, persistent telangiectasia, and/or papulopustular eruptions on the convex areas of the face may be observed [29].

Pathophysiology

Much like in the other causes of BKC, bacteria and their secreted products may play a role in the pathophysiology of rosacea. One study showed that β-hemolytic staphylococcus epidermidis were more likely to be isolated in patients with rosacea than in controls [32]. Furthermore, rosacea is characterized by vasodilation, which leads to increased facial temperature. One study demonstrated that the type and amount of protein secreted by commensal staphylococcal species on the eyelid change with the temperature; at higher temperatures as in with patients with rosacea, the protein profile secreted by *Staphylococcus epidermidis* is distinct from control patients [32]. In another study, patients with ocular rosacea have also been found to have lid margins more likely to be positive for *Staphylococcus aureus*. However, it is important to note that it is unclear whether these positive lid cultures are the cause of the rosacea or a secondary manifestation due to rosacea [33].

More specifically, phlyctenular disease may be associated with rosacea; the conjunctivitis observed in phlyctenular disease is very similar to that observed in ocular rosacea [13]. There may be an association between PKC and rosacea or they may exist as part of the same clinical spectrum [2, 4]. Studies have also shown overlap between patients with PKC and rosacea. In one study of PKC, rosacea dermatitis was present in a subset of patients. Some of those patients demonstrated positivity for *Propionibacterium acnes* on phlyctenule culture and response to tetracycline treatment [4, 5]. Tetracyclines are an effective treatment for both phlyctenular disease and rosacea as well as blepharitis that so often accompanies these two diseases. It is often unknown whether children enrolled in BKC studies developed rosacea later in life. There have been other studies that have similarly identified ocular rosacea in children with PKC as well as positivity on the lids for *Propionibacterium acnes*, though there is no clear link between *Propionibacterium acnes* and the pathogenesis of rosacea [2, 34]. Thus, it is possible that PKC and rosacea exist on a similar spectrum of disease.

Treatment

Basic treatment for ocular rosacea is similar to that discussed for eyelid margin disease and PKC. In adults, the treatment of rosacea is with tetracyclines such as doxycycline. However, this class of drugs is contraindicated in children less than

8 years old. Metronidazole can be an effective option for treating childhood rosacea in those younger than eight for whom tetracyclines are contraindicated [29]. Erythromycin has been used with various levels of success in treating childhood ocular rosacea when tetracyclines cannot be used [28, 29]. Erythromycin can be effective in treating both the dermatologic and ocular components of rosacea. Specifically, it can improve meibomian gland function, improving ocular surface disease.

Conclusion

Eyelid marginal disease, childhood rosacea, and phlyctenular disease are three interrelated conditions that can be manifestations of BKC. They likely encompass a spectrum of the clinical presentation of BKC. Specifically, all three conditions may be related through a shared etiology of staphylococcal hypersensitivity reactions. Treatment relies on eyelid hygiene, management of underlying etiologies with antibacterial medications, and anti-inflammatory therapy. While treatment can be similar for these diseases, there are also disease-specific considerations. More studies are needed to elucidate how these interrelated conditions are part of the same clinical spectrum.

References

1. Hammersmith KM, Cohen EJ, Blake TD, Laibson PR, Rapuano CJ. Blepharokeratoconjuncti vitis in children. Arch Ophthalmol. 2005;123(12):1667–70.
2. Farpour BMD, McClellan KAFF. Diagnosis and management of chronic blepharokeratoconjunctivitis in children. J Pediatr Ophthalmol Strabismus. 2001;38(4):207–12.
3. Gupta N, Dhawan A, Beri S, D'Souza P. Clinical spectrum of pediatric blepharokeratoconjunctivitis. J AAPOS. 2010;14(6):527–9.
4. Culbertson WW, Huang AJ, Mandelbaum SH, Pflugfelder SC, Boozalis GT, Miller D. Effective treatment of phlyctenular keratoconjunctivitis with oral tetracycline. Ophthalmology. 1993;100(9):1358–66.
5. Zaidman GW, Brown SI. Orally administered tetracycline for Phlyctenular keratoconjunctivitis. Am J Ophthalmol. 1981;92(2):178–82.
6. Wu M, Wang X, Han J, Shao T, Wang Y. Evaluation of the ocular surface characteristics and demodex infestation in paediatric and adult blepharokeratoconjunctivitis. BMC Ophthalmol. 2019;19(1):67.
7. Viswalingam M, Rauz S, Morlet N, Dart JK. Blepharokeratoconjunctivitis in children: diagnosis and treatment. Br J Ophthalmol. 2005;89(4):400–3.
8. Meisler DM, Raizman MB, Traboulsi EI. Oral erythromycin treatment for childhood blepharokeratitis. J AAPOS. 2000;4(6):379–80.
9. Jones SM, Weinstein JM, Cumberland P, Klein N, Nischal KK. Visual outcome and corneal changes in children with chronic blepharokeratoconjunctivitis. Ophthalmology. 2007;114(12):2271–80.
10. Singer TR, Isenberg SJ, Apt L. Conjunctival anaerobic and aerobic bacterial flora in paediatric versus adult subjects. Br J Ophthalmol. 1988;72(6):448–51.

11. Luchs J. Azithromycin in DuraSite for the treatment of blepharitis. Clin Ophthalmol. 2010;4:681–8.
12. Donaldson KE, Karp CL, Dunbar MT. Evaluation and treatment of children with ocular rosacea. Cornea. 2007;26(1):42–6.
13. Sorsby A. The Aetiology of Phlyctenular ophthalmia. Br J Ophthalmol. 1942;26(4):159–79.
14. Gautam P, Shrestha GS, Sharma AK. Phlyctenular keratoconjunctivitis among children in the tertiary eye hospital of Kathmandu, Nepal Oman. J Ophthalmol. 2015;8(3):147–50.
15. Thygeson P. The etiology and treatment of phlyctenular keratoconjunctivitis. Am J Ophthalmol. 1951;34(9):1217–36.
16. Rohatgi J, Dhaliwal U. Phlyctenular eye disease: a reappraisal. Jpn J Ophthalmol. 2000;44(2):146–50.
17. Al-Amry MA, Al-Amri A, Khan AO. Resolution of childhood recurrent corneal phlyctenulosis following eradication of an intestinal parasite. J AAPOS. 2008;12(1):89–90.
18. Al-Hussaini MK, Khalifa R, Al-Ansary AT, Hussain GH, Moustafa KM. Phlyctenular eye disease in association with Hymenolepis nana in Egypt. Br J Ophthalmol. 1979;63(9):627–31.
19. Hussein AA, Nasr ME. The role of parasitic infection in the aetiology of phlyctenular eye disease. J Egypt Soc Parasitol. 1991;21(3):865–8.
20. Eleiwa TK, Elmaghrabi A, Helal HG, Abdelrahman SN, ElSheikh RH, Elhusseiny AM. Phlyctenular keratoconjunctivitis in a patient with COVID-19 infection. Cornea. 2021;40(11):1502–4.
21. Ostler HB. Corneal perforation in nontuberculous (staphylococcal) phlyctenular keratoconjunctivitis. Am J Ophthalmol. 1975;79(3):446–8.
22. Blaustein BH, Gurwood AS. Recurrent phlyctenular keratoconjunctivitis: a forme fruste manifestation of rosacea. Optometry. 2001;72(3):179–84.
23. Doan S, Gabison E, Gatinel D, Duong MH, Abitbol O, Hoang-Xuan T. Topical cyclosporine A in severe steroid-dependent childhood phlyctenular keratoconjunctivitis. Am J Ophthalmol. 2006;141(1):62–6.
24. Kymionis GD, Kankariya VP, Kontadakis GA. Tacrolimus ointment 0.03% for treatment of refractory childhood phlyctenular keratoconjunctivitis. Cornea. 2012;31(8):950–2.
25. Yoon CH, Kim MK, Oh JY. Topical tacrolimus 0.03% for maintenance therapy in steroid-dependent, recurrent Phlyctenular keratoconjunctivitis. Cornea. 2018;37(2):168–71.
26. Kroshinsky D, Glick SA. Pediatric rosacea. Dermatol Ther. 2006;19(4):196–201.
27. Doan S, Gabison E, Chiambaretta F, Touati M, Cochereau I. Efficacy of azithromycin 1.5% eye drops in childhood ocular rosacea with phlyctenular blepharokeratoconjunctivitis. J Ophthalmic Inflamm Infect. 2013;3(1):38.
28. Nazir SA, Murphy S, Siatkowski RM, Chodosh J, Siatkowski RL. Ocular rosacea in childhood. Am J Ophthalmol. 2004;137(1):138–44.
29. Chamaillard M, Mortemousque B, Boralevi F, Marques da Costa C, Aitali F, Taïeb A, et al. Cutaneous and ocular signs of childhood rosacea. Arch Dermatol. 2008;144(2):167–71.
30. Marks R, Harcourt-Webster JN. Histopathology of rosacea. Arch Dermatol. 1969;100(6):683–91.
31. Rainer BM, Kang S, Chien AL. Rosacea: epidemiology, pathogenesis, and treatment. Dermatoendocrinol. 2017;9(1):e1361574.
32. Dahl MV, Ross AJ, Schlievert PM. Temperature regulates bacterial protein production: possible role in rosacea. J Am Acad Dermatol. 2004;50(2):266–72.
33. Wise G. Ocular rosacea. Am J Ophthalmol. 1943;26:591–609.
34. Jahns AC, Lundskog B, Dahlberg I, Tamayo NC, McDowell A, Patrick S, et al. No link between rosacea and Propionibacterium acnes. APMIS. 2012;120(11):922–5.

Chapter 3
Allergic and Atopic Disease of the Pediatric Eye

Shudan Wang, Catherine Liu, and Thomas H. Dohlman

Introduction

Allergic and atopic diseases of the eye are among the most common reasons for pediatric ophthalmology referrals. These conditions differ in presentation and severity, but all are rooted in the body's immunologic responses to foreign antigens, particularly type 1 and type 4 hypersensitivity reactions. Addressing these immunologic processes through anti-histamines, mast cell stabilizers, and immunomodulators, along with preventive allergen avoidance measures, is critical to managing the signs and symptoms of allergic disease and avoiding long-term sequelae in these patients. Here we review the pathogenesis, clinical presentation, and therapeutic strategies for the major types of pediatric allergic and atopic eye disease including allergic conjunctivitis, atopic keratoconjunctivitis, vernal keratoconjunctivitis, and giant papillary conjunctivitis.

Allergic Conjunctivitis

Epidemiology

The prevalence of allergic conjunctivitis (AC) is increasing in all populations and is thought to affect up to 25–30% of children [1]. Seasonal/intermittent allergic conjunctivitis (SAC) and perennial/persistent allergic conjunctivitis (PAC) are the most common forms of ocular allergy, affecting approximately 15–20% of the population

S. Wang · C. Liu · T. H. Dohlman (✉)
Cornea Service, Massachusetts Eye and Ear, Department of Ophthalmology, Harvard Medical School, Boston, MA, USA
e-mail: Thomas_Dohlman@meei.harvard.edu

A. Traish, V. P. Douglas (eds.), *Pediatric Ocular Surface Disease*,
https://doi.org/10.1007/978-3-031-30562-7_3

[2]. SAC and PAC can accompany systemic atopy, signs of which include atopic dermatitis, allergic rhinitis, and asthma [3]. SAC is a bilateral acute disease usually caused by environmental allergens and thus is more prevalent from the spring to fall season. In contrast, PAC is a chronic and persistent disease that lasts throughout the year, although it can have periods of exacerbation and remission. PAC is usually due to environmental and household allergens such as animal dander, dust mites, and air pollutants. Around 57% of patients with allergic rhinitis suffer from ocular symptoms, but allergic rhinitis is not a prerequisite for allergic conjunctivitis [4, 5].

Pathophysiology

Seasonal allergic conjunctivitis and perennial allergic conjunctivitis are characterized by a type 1 hypersensitivity reaction [6]. In sensitized individuals, the allergic response is triggered when a specific allergen reaches the conjunctiva and binds mast cell-bound immunoglobulin E (IgE); Th2-cells produce interleukin (IL)-4, IL-5, and IL-13, which induce B cells to produce IgE. Secreted IgE is bound to the surface of mast cells, and when an allergen binds the IgE receptor, an acute reaction is triggered in the form of mast cell degranulation, causing the release of histamine and other preformed inflammatory mediators [4]. These mediators promote the migration and function of various inflammatory cells including eosinophils, neutrophils, basophils, and T lymphocytes in the conjunctival mucosa, a process that occurs over several hours following allergen exposure [7, 8]. Histologically, allergic conjunctivitis is characterized by robust inflammatory cell infiltration of the conjunctiva [9]. As the allergic reaction progresses, increased tear secretion serves to irrigate the ocular surface and carries allergens through the lacrimal ducts into the nasal passage [10].

Clinical Presentation

Seasonal symptoms are triggered by transient allergens such as tree or grass pollens. Perennial symptoms are caused by allergens derived from house dust mites, animal dander, mold spores, cockroaches or rodents, among other sources [11]. However, many patients are polysensitized and can experience perennial symptoms with seasonal exacerbations.

"TIREd" is a mnemonic describing the common signs and symptoms of allergic conjunctivitis: tearing, itching, redness, and edema [2]. Itching is a key symptom of allergic conjunctivitis and may be out of proportion to the degree of hyperemia [12, 13]. Of note, itching is typically worse in the nasal aspect of the conjunctiva [14]. Clinical examination reveals papillary conjunctivitis, and while corneal involvement is rare in SAC and PAC, superficial punctate keratopathy can be present in more severe cases [15]. Conjunctival edema is another characteristic finding of allergic conjunctivitis which can vary from moderate to severe and is sometimes the most prominent feature on examination [13]. The eyelids may be hyperemic and edematous, and this can be more pronounced in the lower eyelid due to gravity. An allergic "shiner," a bluish discoloration of the skin below the eyes, may be present in acute disease as a result of venous congestion [12]. Watery secretions are often noted, and mucous secretions may also be visualized in the tear film [16].

Proper diagnosis of allergic conjunctivitis is made based on history and physical examination, with ocular itching being the most common symptom. Patients may be asymptomatic at the time of presentation, so it is important to ask if their symptoms are worse during a particular season. Inquiring about a family history of atopic disease such as allergic rhinitis, atopic dermatitis, or asthma is important as such a history increases the likelihood of allergic disease. Interestingly, in children, a diagnosis of attention deficit hyperactivity disorder (ADHD) has been associated with a higher likelihood of suffering from allergic conjunctivitis [17]. An allergy consult may be considered when evaluating a patient with allergic conjunctivitis, and allergy evaluation may entail allergen skin prick-testing, which has high test sensitivity [18].

Management

Allergen avoidance is the foundation of allergic conjunctivitis management. To minimize allergen exposure, patients should be encouraged to wash their hands frequently and avoid touching or rubbing their eyes. Exposure can be reduced by keeping windows closed, using screen filters and air conditioners and increasing patient awareness of local pollen count monitoring in order to minimize unnecessary exposures [12]. Strategies to reduce exposure to animals may include removing pets from the home, although this recommendation can be understandably challenging for many families [19]. House dust mite control measures include maintaining humidity in the home between 35% and 50%, using mite-proof covers for bedding, washing, bedding weekly and use of a central ventilation system with adequate filtration or vents to the outside [19]. Large wraparound sunglasses can be used to reduce contact with allergens and reduce photophobia [20]. Cold compresses and cold artificial tears or ointments are useful adjunctive therapies in allergic conjunctivitis as they relieve allergic symptoms and reduce allergen concentration, especially in acute allergic conjunctivitis [4]. Recent work has demonstrated that cold compresses and artificial tears can have an additive effect on the pharmacology of topical anti-allergy agents [21].

Topical anti-histamines, mast cell stabilizers, and dual-action (combined antihistamine and mast cell stabilizer) drugs are the first-choice pharmacologic treatments for allergic conjunctivitis [17]. There are many commercially available topical anti-histamine agents, the most frequently used being azelastine, levocabastine, and pheniramine maleate, with a frequency of 2–4 times/day [12]. Oral antihistamines are effective in cases of allergic conjunctivitis, however, they have a higher frequency of systemic side effects, such as somnolence, than topical antihistamines [17, 21]. Epinastine and olopatadine-eluting contact lenses have been produced and may act as both a physical allergen barrier and sustained-release delivery device [8]. Mast cell stabilizers inhibit mast cell degranulation and are therefore useful as a prophylactic strategy, with a necessary loading period of around 2 weeks (i.e., pre-treatment with a mast cell stabilizer prior to allergy season). Mast cell stabilizers include drugs such as cromolyn sodium, nedocromil sodium, lodoxamide, pemirolast [17]. They all require a preloading period and frequent installation (3–4 times/day), [17]. Combined anti-histamine and mast cell stabilizer agents are also available and compared to single-mechanism anti-histamines and mast cell stabilizers, these dual-activity agents are clinically superior in both symptom relief and tolerability [6]. Such agents include bepotastine, epinastine, azelastine, alcaftadine, ketotifen, and olopatadine, making twice daily dosing possible [17].

NSAIDs can decrease symptoms in allergic conjunctivitis but patients sometimes report a stinging/burning sensation when instilled and in general their use is not widespread in this condition [21]. Ketorolac tromethamine 0.5% is the only ophthalmic NSAID currently approved by the FDA for the relief of ocular itching in seasonal allergic conjunctivitis with a suggested dose of 4 times/day [22]. When used, topical NSAIDs are often used in addition to a topical anti-histamine or dual-action agent [17]. NSAIDs can have adverse effects including corneal ulceration and corneal perforation and as such their use should be extremely limited in the allergic setting [21]. Although effective, topical and intranasal steroids are not usually required for the management of PAC and SAC. Intranasal steroids are effective in reducing the nasal and ocular symptoms of SAC and PAC in part because ocular symptoms may be due to a nasal-ocular reflex [17, 21]. Any use of steroid agents must take into account the risk of their well-known adverse effects, which include ocular hypertension and cataract formation [23].

Alpha-adrenergic agonists were among the first topical treatments to be approved for the treatment of allergic symptoms. They are sold over the counter and are used to counteract hyperemia but are not recommended in adolescents and children. They have a short duration and have many adverse effects including tachyphylaxis, ocular irritation, and hypersensitivity [21]. They may also lead to rebound hyperemia and symptoms. Due to the risk-benefit ratio, alpha-adrenergic agonists are generally discouraged in the management of allergic conjunctivitis.

Vernal Keratoconjunctivitis

Epidemiology

Vernal keratoconjunctivitis (VKC) typically begins in the first decade of life and generally resolves spontaneously after puberty, although in the most severe cases, it may leave permanent damage to cornea and conjunctiva [24]. VKC affects males more frequently than females, with a ratio of 2–3:1. It is usually observed in tropical climates, including in Mediterranean countries, the Middle East, Central and West Africa, India, and South America, but it can also be observed less frequently in colder climates [13, 24]. It often presents seasonally, with a maximum incidence at the end of spring and summer, suggesting a hypersensitivity reaction to environmental allergens. However, there may also be symptoms throughout the year, especially in warmer climates where the condition can become perennial [25]. Fifteen to 60% of affected children may also present with other atopic diseases [26] and interestingly, children with VKC have been shown to have a higher incidence of immunoglobulin deficiency and vitamin D deficiency [27, 28].

Pathophysiology

The development of VKC is likely multifactorial and is thought to be the result of interactions between various immunologic, genetic, and environmental factors such as sunlight and wind exposure [13, 14, 22]. The association of VKC with specific HLA haplotypes has been investigated with inconsistent results [29], and the ocular surface microbiome has also been implicated in disease pathogenesis [25].

VKC involves IgE-mediated, Th1-mediated, and Th2-mediated immunoinflammatory mechanisms and is considered both a type 1 and type 4 hypersensitivity reaction [29]. VKC patients overexpress both Th1 and Th2-associated cytokines, pro-inflammatory molecules, chemokines, and growth factors [29]. VKC and allergic conjunctivitis may have some overlap and they are not mutually exclusive, with about half of VKC patients also experiencing allergic conjunctivitis, with more severe ocular symptoms upon allergen exposure [30]. Allergen-specific IgE has been detected in both the serum and tears of VKC patients, at least in the active phase of the disease. VKC is also thought to represent a link between atopy and systemic autoimmunity, as it has been reported that 31% of children with VKC have antinuclear antibodies and about 50% have a family history of autoimmune disorders [31, 32].

Clinical Presentation

Typical manifestations of VKC include itching, redness, and watery or mucous discharge, as in other forms of ocular allergy, in addition to photophobia and foreign body sensation. Usually, the lid margins are not involved, a finding which can be useful for diagnosis [27]. VKC is classified clinically as tarsal, limbal, or mixed; the tarsal form is more frequent in Europe and the Americas, while the limbal type is the predominant form of presentation in Africa [33]. In the tarsal form, giant papillae appear in the tarsal conjunctiva (Fig. 3.1) and can increase in size with time to become "cobblestone-like" papillae, often surrounded by mucus collections [25, 27]. In the limbal form, rounded nodules formed by lymphocytic infiltrates are observed at the limbus. At their vertex are collections of necrotic eosinophils, neutrophils, and mast cells that appear as white dots which are clinically referred to as Horner-Trantas dots [27]. These dots normally appear when VKC is active and disappear between active episodes [25]. The mixed form of VKC shows both tarsal and

Fig. 3.1 Photograph of the tarsal conjunctiva in a child with active vernal keratoconjunctivitis illustrating large papillae

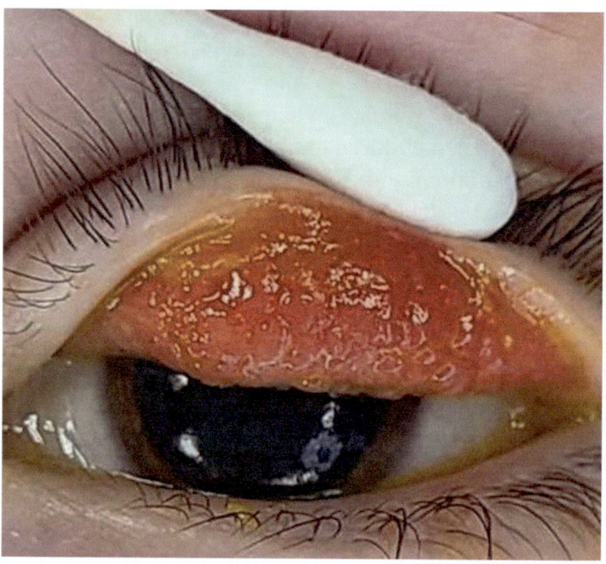

limbal papillae. VKC can be complicated by punctate keratopathy that usually starts in the superior cornea and may evolve to form plaque or shield ulcers that can present as subepithelial white plaques [13, 34]. Other possible sequelae of VKC include corneal scarring, limbal stem cell deficiency, and amblyopia [35].

Management

As in allergic conjunctivitis, allergen avoidance is important, and cold compresses and artificial tears may help to alleviate symptoms in mild cases or can serve as an adjunctive therapy to pharmacologic treatment [25]. First-line pharmacologic therapy for VKC consists of topical treatment with mast cell stabilizers, anti-histamines, and steroids. Mast cell stabilizers are the mainstay of prophylaxis. In milder cases, anti-histamines may be of benefit, but more severe cases often require corticosteroids which are then tapered according to the clinical response. NSAIDs may be used in conjunction with other topical anti-inflammatory medications to provide rapid relief of symptoms [35], but these agents can cause corneal complications as discussed above and their use should be limited [21]. Topical corticosteroids are a critical component of VKC management, particularly in VKC exacerbations. Broadly, there are two treatment regimens: pulsed and prolonged treatment. Pulsed therapy consists of administration 3–4 times a day for 3–5 days and is frequently used for VKC and AKC. Prolonged therapy consists of administration 3–4 times a day for 1–3 weeks followed by slow tapering, which may be used occasionally in severe chronic forms of disease [36].

To avoid known adverse effects of steroids, other non-steroid immunomodulatory treatments, particularly calcineurin inhibitors, are often employed. Cyclosporine A is a calcineurin inhibitor that inhibits T cell activation and function. It also has inhibitory effects on eosinophil and mast cell activation [37]. Low-dose cyclosporine has emerged as an attractive alternative to corticosteroids in VKC. It generally has a favorable adverse effect profile, with burning upon instillation being the most common reported symptom [38]. Topical 0.05% cyclosporine A, which is commercially available, has been used in various regimens, including one regimen reported as 6x/day for 2 weeks followed by tapering to 4 times a day has been shown to improve clinical signs and symptoms of VKC, as well as decrease tear cytokine concentration [39].

Tacrolimus is another calcineurin inhibitor that acts to inhibit T cell activation and prevent the release of inflammatory cytokines [40]. Tacrolimus drops are not commercially available in the United States but can be compounded, and tacrolimus ointment is commonly used off-label in the eye [41]. Recent studies suggest that tacrolimus may be similar, or even superior to, cyclosporine A in the treatment of VKC [39].

Recalcitrant cases of VKC may require treatment with systemic medications, including oral corticosteroids or other immunomodulatory agents. Corneal complications such as non-healing shield ulcers (Fig. 3.2) or corneal plaques may require surgical intervention. These treatments may range from scraping/debridement to superficial keratectomy. In rare cases of refractory giant papillae unresponsive to medical therapy, surgical interventions such as cryoablation may be employed. Amniotic membrane transplantation may be necessary to treat epithelial lesions and ulcers in refractory cases [42].

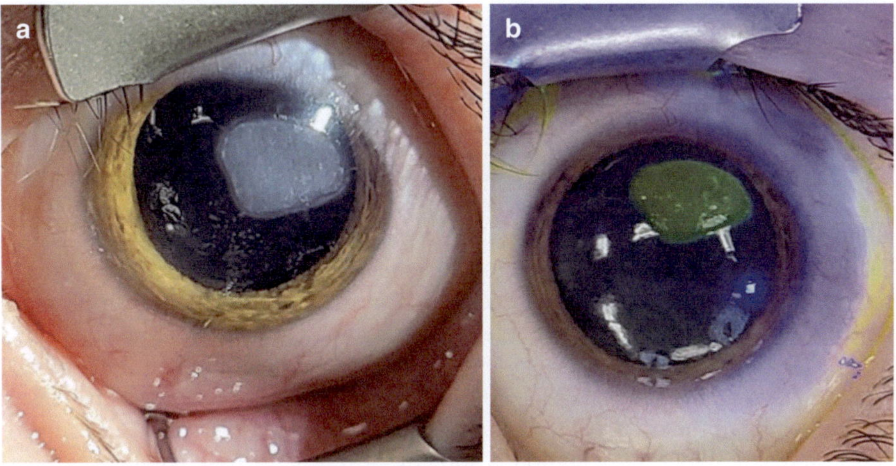

Fig. 3.2 (**a** and **b**) Photographs of a shield ulcer in a child with active vernal keratoconjunctivitis [**a** (left); without stain, **b** (right); with stain]

Atopic Keratoconjunctivitis

Epidemiology

Atopic keratoconjunctivitis (AKC) is more frequent in males and can present as early as the first decade of life, with a peak presentation between the ages of 20 and 50. AKC is associated with a family history of atopy, along with a personal history of atopic dermatitis or other allergic diseases such as eczema, asthma, and urticaria [43]. The percentage of patients with atopic dermatitis who develop AKC ranges from 25% to 42% [44].

Of note, the first FDA approved biologic systemic therapy for atopic dermatitis, dupilumab (Dupixent®, Regeneron & Sanofi, USA) has been associated with a higher incidence of conjunctivitis than the natural occurrence among the comorbid conditions. Ocular presentations may range from mild to severe involving primarily the conjunctiva and cornea. Therefore it is critical that ophthalmic providers consider this on the differential among their pediatric patients and in particular review systemic medication history [45].

Pathophysiology

AKC is both a type 1 and a type 4 hypersensitivity immune reaction, with the predominant effector cells being both Th1 and Th2 cells, both of which are a potent source of cytokines and chemokines and stimulate eosinophil production [46]. AKC is also considered to be, at least in part, an IgE-dependent mechanism [15]. However, in one study, 45% of the patients with AKC did not display a hypersensitivity reaction to common allergens [13].

Clinical Presentation

Like VKC, AKC can be considered an ocular manifestation of atopic dermatitis and is the most severe form of chronic allergic conjunctivitis. It is a bilateral inflammatory chronic keratoconjunctivitis that affects not only the ocular surface but also the eyelids and is sometimes considered to be a form of blepharokerato-conjunctivitis. Patients report intense itching most of the year that can be more severe during the winter and in colder climates [43]. Other presenting symptoms include ocular pain, erythema, ropy or mucoid discharge, tearing, burning, photophobia, and visual disturbances [41]. On examination, signs of AKC can be classified according to the involved tissue, namely the eyelids, conjunctiva, and cornea. Periorbital skin hyperpigmentation is sometimes referred to as "panda eyes," and lid thickening and edema can cause formation of linear lid creases known as Dennie-Morgan lines. Patients can also develop Hertoghe's sign, which is thinning of the lateral aspect of the eyebrows. More advanced chronic disease may also cause keratinization of the eyelid margins, blepharitis, madarosis, eyelid deformities, and reactive ptosis. Chronic inflammation of the tarsal and forniceal conjunctiva leads to conjunctival thickening, hyperemia, chemosis, and papillary hypertrophy. Papillae are often observed on the upper and lower tarsal conjunctiva. In later stages, the papillae can be replaced by diffuse conjunctival scarring, leading to forniceal foreshortening and symblepharon. Limbal Horner-Trantas dots can be observed as well, especially during seasonal exacerbations [45]. Corneal involvement appears to be secondary to conjunctival and eyelid pathology and may vary from superficial punctate keratitis to corneal ulcers, corneal scarring, and pannus [47]. Chronic AKC can be associated with a number of other complications including staphylococcal blepharoconjunctivitis, cataracts, and limbal stem cell deficiency [15].

Management

The treatment of AKC is focused on managing acute flares as well as the underlying disease process, with a goal of decreasing symptoms and preventing permanent, vision-threatening complications. Topical anti-histamines and mast cell stabilizers used in allergic conjunctivitis are usually less effective in AKC, but many of the treatment principles utilized for VKC can be applied to AKC. For AKC of any severity level, topical or systemic corticosteroids can be used to control inflammation, usually 3–4 times a day for 1–3 weeks with an appropriate taper whenever possible. Given the pathophysiology of AKC, T cell modulation is a favored therapeutic approach, and the calcineurin inhibitors cyclosporine A and tacrolimus are commonly used. Randomized control trials have shown that topical 0.05% cyclosporine A four times a day is safe and effective in improving both signs and symptoms in mild as well as refractory cases of AKC [48, 49]. Topical tacrolimus has also been shown to reduce signs and symptoms of AKC, both as a 0.1% solution and a 0.03% ointment twice a day [50, 51]. AKC complicated by subcapsular cataracts or severe ocular surface disease may require surgical interventions such as superficial keratectomy and cataract surgery, respectively, or more involved procedures such as limbal stem cell transplantation or even keratoprosthesis implantation [52]. Onset of dupilumab-associated conjunctivitis during trials correlated with more severe atopic dermatitis at baseline. The conjunctivitis was found to respond to a similar management approach as the non-drug induced forms of atopic eye disease as described above. In severe cases, the cessation of dupilumab therapy may be warranted to control the ocular inflammation [53].

Giant Papillary Conjunctivitis

Epidemiology

Giant papillary conjunctivitis (GPC) is an immunoinflammatory disorder that has features of allergic and atopic disease. Although GPC is most commonly associated with contact lens wear, it may also occur in the setting of ocular prosthetics, exposed sutures or scleral buckles, glaucoma filtering blebs, and band keratopathy, among other conditions [54]. The incidence of GPC appears to be influenced by the frequency of contact lens replacement, type of contact lens, increased wearing time, poor contact lens hygiene, increased lens size, and poor lens fit [55]. It appears that there is a shorter time to onset of GPC in soft contact lens wearers compared to rigid contact lens wearers, as one report showed that the average time to GPC onset following contact lens initiation was 10 months with soft contacts, compared to a range of 14 months to 9 years with hard contacts [56]. GPC and atopy may be closely related as the signs and symptoms of GPC are more severe in atopic patients as compared to non-atopic patients [51] and there is a correlation between seasonal onset of allergies and GPC [57].

Pathophysiology

The exact pathophysiology of GPC is not well understood and is likely multifactorial, [50] involving nonspecific foreign body and mechanical trauma responses, as well as immediate (type 1) and delayed (type 4) hypersensitivity reactions [58]. As described above, as part of a type 1 hypersensitivity reaction, conjunctival mast cells bound by IgE mount a nonspecific degranulating response upon antigen exposure. This is followed by tissue inflammation and further infiltration of inflammatory cells, including mast cells, eosinophils, and basophils [59]. In patients with bilateral GPC but asymmetric eye symptomatology, the expression of IgE has been reported to be higher in the more symptomatic eye [60]. Conjunctival stromal fibrosis and decreased conjunctival cellularity can develop in patients with chronic GPC [61], and M cells (membranous epithelial cells) in the conjunctiva-associated lymphoid tissue of patients with GPC have been reported [62]. The presence of these M cells, which are normally involved in upregulating immune responses through the uptake and transport of antigens to immune cells, further supports an immunologic basis for GPC [58].

Clinical Presentation

The symptoms of GPC include itching, foreign body sensation, watery or mucous discharge, and decreased contact lens tolerance. Signs of GPC include excess mucus production, hyperemia, conjunctival opacification, and multiple giant papillae that can be highlighted by fluorescein staining [54]. Larger papillae often have overlying white "caps" that regress as the condition improves and are likely inflammatory infiltrates in the conjunctival epithelium [54]. Although signs and symptoms are usually present bilaterally, one study found that 10% of GPC cases were unilateral [56]. In those individuals developing GPC due to contact use, the characteristics of the papillae may vary by the type of contact lens worn; in one report the authors observed that the papillae associated with soft contact lens wear progressed from small clusters to elevated, giant papillae with a flattening of the top surface and a "mushroom" appearance [52]. In terms of distribution, papillae are usually initially located in the superior tarsal conjunctiva along the upper tarsal border, with subsequent spread to surrounding regions [52]. In rigid contact lens wearers, papillae can be seen in the central area of the tarsal plate and along the lid margin [63]. In cases of GPC attributed to exposed sutures, filtering blebs, and elevated band keratopathy, papillae have been noted to localize in the region of the superior tarsal conjunctiva directly overlying the inciting pathology [54]. Cases of GPC attributed to scleral lenses or prosthetic shells are often characterized by papillae on the tarsal surface and in the superior fornix [54]. Corneal complications are relatively rare in GPC, but superficial punctate keratitis and shield ulcers may occur [64].

Management

Since contact lens wear is often responsible for the initial trauma and inflammatory response in most cases of GPC, temporary contact lens wear discontinuation is the first step in management [65]. Discontinuation of contact lens wear is recommended for 2–4 weeks, or until signs and symptoms resolve [54]. Following this period, if possible, eye care providers should refit the patient with either daily disposable soft contact lenses or soft contact lenses that are replaced every 1–2 weeks [54]. In order to achieve safe and uncomplicated contact lens wear, it is important for patients to adhere to regular and effective contact lens hygiene practice. A switch from soft contact lenses to rigid gas-permeable contact lenses may also be considered if other measures have failed to improve the signs and symptoms of GPC [54]. As described above, anti-allergy therapies are often used to treat GPC during the temporary contact lens holiday [63]. These therapies include anti-histamine agents, mast cell stabilizers, or dual-acting agents, 2–4 times a day. When anti-allergy medications do not sufficiently improve symptoms, and/or in severe cases of GPC, corticosteroid eye drops are employed [62]. Topical NSAIDs four times a day may also be used as an adjunct to steroids in individuals with uncontrolled GPC, or as an alternate therapy in individuals with adverse effects to steroids [22]. In rare instances where signs and symptoms of GPC persist despite the above-mentioned management, patients with GPC may require other immunomodulatory therapies. Kymionis et al. reported a refractory case of GPC that resolved after 1 month of tacrolimus 0.03% ointment twice a day [66]. The case described had not responded to anti-histamines, mast cell stabilizers, topical corticosteroids, or surgical resection/cryopexy. Moreover, there are multiple reports on the safety and efficacy of topical tacrolimus and cyclosporine A in the treatment of giant papillae associated with vernal keratoconjunctivitis

[39]. On rare occasions, surgical interventions may be needed for severe, refractory cases of GPC. These procedures include cryotherapy of papillae and excision of papillae followed by transplantation of amniotic membrane, autologous conjunctival grafts, or oral mucosal grafts to cover the resulting tarsal defects [67].

Conclusion

Allergic and atopic eye diseases are extremely common causes of ocular morbidity in the pediatric population. In the present review, we have discussed the prevalence, diagnosis, pathophysiology, and management of these conditions. With careful clinical consideration and a stepwise approach to treatment, the symptoms and signs of allergic eye disease can be effectively managed to improve quality of life and minimize long-term sequelae in these children. We look forward to a deeper understanding of the underlying mechanisms in allergic eye disease and development of novel therapeutic strategies for these conditions in the future.

Conflicts of Interest None of the authors have any relevant conflicts of interest to disclose.

References

1. Fauquert JL. Diagnosing and managing allergic conjunctivitis in childhood: the allergist's perspective. Pediatr Allergy Immunol. 2019;30(4):405–14. https://doi.org/10.1111/pai.13035.
2. Wong AH, Barg SS, Leung AK. Seasonal and perennial allergic conjunctivitis. Recent Pat Inflamm Allergy Drug Discov. 2009;3(2):118–27. https://doi.org/10.2174/187221309788489733.
3. O'Brien TP. Allergic conjunctivitis: an update on diagnosis and management. Curr Opin Allergy Clin Immunol. 2013;13(5):543–9. https://doi.org/10.1097/ACI.0b013e328364ec3a.
4. Canonica GW, Bousquet J, Mullol J, Scadding GK, Virchow JC. A survey of the burden of allergic rhinitis in Europe. Allergy. 2007;62:17–25. https://doi.org/10.1111/j.1398-9995.2007.01549.x.
5. Roberts G, Pfaar O, Akdis CA, Ansotegui IJ, Durham SR, Gerth van Wijk R, Halken S, Larenas-Linnemann D, Pawankar R, Pitsios C, Sheikh A. EAACI guidelines on allergen immunotherapy: allergic rhinoconjunctivitis. Allergy. 2018;73(4):765–98. https://doi.org/10.1111/all.13317.
6. Dupuis P, Prokopich CL, Hynes A, Kim H. A contemporary look at allergic conjunctivitis. Allergy Asthma Clin Immunol. 2020;16(1):1–8. https://doi.org/10.1186/s13223-020-0403-9.
7. Leonardi A, De Dominicis C, Motterle L. Immunopathogenesis of ocular allergy: a schematic approach to different clinical entities. Curr Opin Allergy Clin Immunol. 2007;7(5):429–35. https://doi.org/10.1097/ACI.0b013e3282ef8674.
8. Bielory L, Schoenberg D. Emerging therapeutics for ocular surface disease. Curr Allergy Asthma Rep. 2019;19:16. https://doi.org/10.1007/s11882-019-0844-8.
9. Bielory L. Allergic and immunologic disorders of the eye. Part II: ocular allergy. J Allergy Clin Immunol. 2000;106(6):1019–32. https://doi.org/10.1067/mai.2000.111238.
10. Prokopich CL, Lee-Poy M, Kim H. Interprofessional management of allergic conjunctivitis: a proposed algorithm for Canadian clinical practice. Can J Optom. 2018;80(3):11–27. https://doi.org/10.15353/cjo.80.257.

11. Bielory L, Meltzer EO, Nichols KK, Melton R, Thomas RK, Bartlett JD. An algorithm for the management of allergic conjunctivitis. Allergy Asthma Proc. 2013;34(5):408–20. https://doi.org/10.2500/aap.2013.34.3695.

12. La Rosa M, Lionetti E, Reibaldi M, Russo A, Longo A, Leonardi S, Tomarchio S, Avitabile T, Reibaldi A. Allergic conjunctivitis: a comprehensive review of the literature. Ital J Pediatr. 2013;39:1–8. https://doi.org/10.1186/1824-7288-39-18.

13. Foster CS. The pathophysiology of ocular allergy: current thinking. Allergy. 1995;50:6–9. https://doi.org/10.1111/j.1398-9995.1995.tb04250.x.

14. Berger WE, Granet DB, Kabat AG. Diagnosis and management of allergic conjunctivitis in pediatric patients. Allergy Asthma Proc. 2017;38(1) https://doi.org/10.2500/aap.2017.38.4003.

15. Fauquert JL, Jedrzejczak-Czechowicz M, Rondon C, Calder V, Silva D, Kvenshagen BK, Callebaut I, Allegri P, Santos N, Doan S, Perez FD. Conjunctival allergen provocation test: guidelines for daily practice. Allergy. 2017;72(1):43–54. https://doi.org/10.1111/all.12986.

16. Varu DM, Rhee MK, Akpek EK, Amescua G, Farid M, Garcia-Ferrer FJ, Lin A, Musch DC, Mah FS, Dunn SP. Conjunctivitis preferred practice pattern®. Ophthalmology. 2019;126(1):P94–169. https://doi.org/10.1016/j.ophtha.2018.10.020.

17. Miyazaki C, Koyama M, Ota E, Swa T, Mlunde LB, Amiya RM, Tachibana Y, Yamamoto-Hanada K, Mori R. Allergic diseases in children with attention deficit hyperactivity disorder: a systematic review and meta-analysis. BMC Psychiatry. 2017;17:1–2. https://doi.org/10.1186/s12888-017-1281-7.

18. Bernstein IL, Li JT, Bernstein DI, Hamilton R, Spector SL, Tan R, Sicherer S, Golden DB, Khan DA, Nicklas RA, Portnoy JM. Allergy diagnostic testing: an updated practice parameter. Ann Allergy Asthma Immunol. 2008;100(3):S1–48. https://doi.org/10.1016/S1081-1206(10)60305-5.

19. Portnoy J, Miller JD, Williams PB, Chew GL, Miller JD, Zaitoun F, Phipatanakul W, Kennedy K, Barnes C, Grimes C, Larenas-Linnemann D. Environmental assessment and exposure control of dust mites: a practice parameter. Ann Allergy Asthma Immunol. 2013;111(6):465–507. https://doi.org/10.1016/j.anai.2013.09.018.

20. Sánchez-Hernández MC, Montero J, Rondon C, Benitez del Castillo JM, Velázquez E, Herreras JM, Fernández-Parra B, Merayo-Lloves J, Del Cuvillo A, Vega F, Valero A. Consensus document on allergic conjunctivitis (DECA). J Investig Allergol Clin Immunol. 2015;

21. Leonardi A, Bogacka E, Fauquert JL, Kowalski ML, Groblewska A, Jedrzejczak-Czechowicz M, Doan S, Marmouz F, Demoly P, Delgado L. Ocular allergy: recognizing and diagnosing hypersensitivity disorders of the ocular surface. Allergy 2012 ;67(11):1327-1337. https://doi.org/10.1111/all.12009

22. Kaufman AR. Allergic eye disease. Pediatr Clin North Am. 2014;61(3):607–20. https://doi.org/10.1016/j.pcl.2014.03.009.

23. Gaballa SA, Kompella UB, Elgarhy O, Alqahtani AM, Pierscionek B, Alany RG, Abdelkader H. Corticosteroids in ophthalmology: drug delivery innovations, pharmacology, clinical applications, and future perspectives. Drug Deliv Transl Res. 2021;11:866–93. https://doi.org/10.1007/s13346-020-00843-z.

24. Zicari AM, Nebbioso M, Lollobrigida V, Bardanzellu F, Celani C, Occasi F, Cesoni Marcelli A, Duse M. Vernal keratoconjunctivitis: atopy and autoimmunity. Eur Rev Med Pharmacol Sci. 2013;17(10):1419–23.

25. Addis H, Jeng BH. Vernal keratoconjunctivitis. Clin Ophthalmol. 12:119–23. https://doi.org/10.2147/OPTH.S129552.

26. De Smedt S, Wildner G, Kestelyn P. Vernal keratoconjunctivitis: an update. Br J Ophthalmol. 2013;97(1):9–14. https://doi.org/10.1136/bjophthalmol-2011-301376.

27. Bozkurt B, Artac H, Ozdemir H, Ünlü A, Bozkurt MK, Irkec M. Serum vitamin D levels in children with vernal keratoconjunctivitis. Ocul Immunol Inflamm. 2018;26(3):435–9. https://doi.org/10.1080/09273948.2016.1235714.

28. Bozkurt B, Artac H, Arslan N, Gokturk B, Bozkurt MK, Reisli I, Irkec M. Systemic atopy and immunoglobulin deficiency in Turkish patients with vernal keratoconjunctivitis. Ocul Immunol Inflamm. 2013;21(1):28–33. https://doi.org/10.3109/09273948.2012.723110.

29. Tesse R, Spadavecchia L, Fanelli P, Paglialunga C, Capozza M, Favoino B, Armenio L, Cavallo L. New insights into childhood Vernal keratoconjunctivitis-associated factors. Pediatr Allergy Immunol. 2012;23(7):682–5. https://doi.org/10.1111/j.1399-3038.2012.01281.x.

30. Sacchetti M, Abicca I, Bruscolini A, Cavaliere C, Nebbioso M, Lambiase A. Allergic conjunctivitis: current concepts on pathogenesis and management. J Biol Regul Homeost Agents. 2018;32(1 Suppl. 1):49–60.

31. Zicari AM, Capata G, Nebbioso M, De Castro G, Midulla F, Leonardi L, Loffredo L, Spalice A, Perri L, Duse M. Vernal Keratoconjunctivitis: an update focused on clinical grading system. Ital J Pediatr. 2019;45:1–6. https://doi.org/10.1186/s13052-019-0656-4.

32. Occasi F, Zicari AM, Petrarca L, Nebbioso M, Salvatori G, Duse M. Vernal Keratoconjunctivitis and immune-mediated diseases: One unique way to symptom control? Pediatr Allergy Immunol. 2015;26(3):289–91. https://doi.org/10.1111/pai.12350.

33. Bonini S. Allergy and the eye. Chem Immunol Allergy. 2014;100:105–8. https://doi.org/10.1159/000358615.

34. Solomon A. Corneal complications of vernal keratoconjunctivitis. Curr Opin Allergy Clin Immunol. 2015;15(5):489–94. https://doi.org/10.1097/ACI.0000000000000202.

35. Kosrirukvongs P, Luengchaichawange C. Topical cyclosporine 0.5 per cent and preservative-free ketorolac tromethamine 0.5 per cent in vernal keratoconjunctivitis. J Med Assoc Thai. 2004;87(2):190–7.

36. Villegas BV, Benitez-del-Castillo JM. Current knowledge in allergic conjunctivitis. Turk J Ophthalmol. 2021;51(1):45. https://doi.org/10.4274/tjo.galenos.2020.11456.

37. Donnenfeld E, Pflugfelder SC. Topical ophthalmic cyclosporine: pharmacology and clinical uses. Surv Ophthalmol. 2009;54(3):321–38. https://doi.org/10.1016/j.survophthal.2009.02.002.

38. Pucci N, Caputo R, Mori F, De Libero C, Di Grande L, Massai C, Bernardini R, Novembre E. Long-term safety and efficacy of topical cyclosporine in 156 children with vernal keratoconjunctivitis. Int J Immunopathol Pharmacol. 2010;23(3):865–71. https://doi.org/10.1177/039463201002300322.

39. Oray M, Toker E. Tear cytokine levels in vernal keratoconjunctivitis: the effect of topical 0.05% cyclosporine a therapy. Cornea. 2013;32(8):1149–54. https://doi.org/10.1097/ICO.0b013e31828ffdf8.

40. Zhai J, Gu J, Yuan J, Chen J. Tacrolimus in the treatment of ocular diseases. BioDrugs. 2011;25:89–103. https://doi.org/10.2165/11587010-000000000-00000.

41. Vichyanond P, Kosrirukvongs P. Use of cyclosporine A and tacrolimus in treatment of vernal keratoconjunctivitis. Curr Allergy Asthma Rep. 2013 Jun;13:308–14. https://doi.org/10.1007/s11882-013-0345-0.

42. Guo P, Kheirkhah A, Zhou WW, Qin L, Shen XL. Surgical resection and amniotic membrane transplantation for treatment of refractory giant papillae in vernal keratoconjunctivitis. Cornea. 2013;32(6):816–20. https://doi.org/10.1097/ICO.0b013e31826a1e53.

43. Patel N, Venkateswaran N, Wang Z, Galor A. Ocular involvement in atopic disease: a review. Curr Opin Ophthalmol. 2018;29(6):576–81. https://doi.org/10.1097/ICU.0000000000000532.

44. Zhan H, Smith L, Calder V, Buckley R, Lightman S. Clinical and immunological features of atopic keratoconjunctivitis. Int Ophthalmol Clin. 2003;43(1):59–71. https://doi.org/10.1097/00004397-200343010-00008.

45. Bansal A, Simpson EL, Paller AS, Siegfried EC, Blauvelt A, de Bruin-Weller M, Corren J, Sher L, Guttman-Yassky E, Chen Z, Daizadeh N. Conjunctivitis in dupilumab clinical trials for adolescents with atopic dermatitis or asthma. Am J Clin Dermatol. 2021;22:101–15. https://doi.org/10.1007/s40257-020-00577-1.

46. Ridolo E, Kihlgren P, Pellicelli I, Nizi MC, Pucciarini F, Incorvaia C. Atopic keratoconjunctivitis: pharmacotherapy for the elderly. Drugs Aging. 2019;(36):581–8. https://doi.org/10.1007/s40266-019-00676-7.

47. Power WJ, Tugal-Tutkun I, Foster CS. Long-term follow-up of patients with atopic keratoconjunctivitis. Ophthalmology. 1998;105(4):637–42. https://doi.org/10.1016/S0161-6420(98)94017-9.
48. Daniell M, Constantinou M, Vu HT, Taylor HR. Randomised controlled trial of topical ciclosporin A in steroid dependent allergic conjunctivitis. Br J Ophthalmol. 2006;90(4):461–4. https://doi.org/10.1136/bjo.2005.082461.
49. Akpek EK, Dart JK, Watson S, Christen W, Dursun D, Yoo S, O'Brien TP, Schein OD, Gottsch JD. A randomized trial of topical cyclosporin 0.05% in topical steroid–resistant atopic keratoconjunctivitis. Ophthalmology. 2004;111(3):476–82. https://doi.org/10.1016/j.ophtha.2003.05.035.
50. Yazu H, Fukagawa K, Shimizu E, Sato Y, Fujishima H. Long-term outcomes of 0.1% tacrolimus eye drops in eyes with severe allergic conjunctival diseases. Allergy Asthma Clin Immunol. 2021;17(1):1–9. https://doi.org/10.1186/s13223-021-00513-w.
51. Tzu JH, Utine CA, Stern ME, Akpek EK. Topical calcineurin inhibitors in the treatment of steroid-dependent atopic keratoconjunctivitis. Cornea. 2012;31(6):649–54. https://doi.org/10.1097/ICO.0b013e31822481c2.
52. Jabbehdari S, Starnes TW, Kurji KH, Eslani M, Cortina MS, Holland EJ, Djalilian AR. Management of advanced ocular surface disease in patients with severe atopic keratoconjunctivitis. Ocul Surf. 2019;17(2):303–9. https://doi.org/10.1016/j.jtos.2018.12.002.
53. Akinlade B, Guttman-Yassky E, Bruin-Weller M, Simpson EL, Blauvelt A, Cork MJ, Prens E, Asbell P, Akpek E, Corren J, Bachert C. Conjunctivitis in dupilumab clinical trials. Br J Dermatol. 2019;181(3):459–73. https://doi.org/10.1111/bjd.17869.
54. Donshik PC, Ehlers WH, Ballow M. Giant papillary conjunctivitis. Immunol Allergy Clin North Am. 2008;28(1):83–103. https://doi.org/10.1016/j.iac.2007.11.001.
55. Kenny SE, Tye CB, Johnson DA, Kheirkhah A. Giant papillary conjunctivitis: a review. Ocul Surf. 2020;18(3):396–402. https://doi.org/10.1016/j.jtos.2020.03.007.
56. Allansmith MR, Korb DR, Greiner JV, Henriquez AS, Simon MA, Finnemore VM. Giant papillary conjunctivitis in contact lens wearers. Am J Ophthalmol. 1977;83(5):697–708. https://doi.org/10.1016/0002-9394(77)90137-4.
57. Begley CG, Riggle AN, Tuel JA. Association of giant papillary conjunctivitis with seasonal allergies. Optom Vis Sci. 1990;67(3):192–5. https://doi.org/10.1097/00006324-199003000-00008.
58. Richmond PP. Giant papillary conjunctivitis: an overview. J Am Optom Assoc. 1979;50(3):343–7.
59. National Research Council, Working Group on Contact Lens Use Under Adverse Conditions. Considerations in contact lens use under adverse conditions: proceedings of a symposium. https://doi.org/10.17226/1773
60. Fukagawa K, Saito H, Azuma N, Tsubota K, Iikura Y, Oguchi Y. Histamine and tryptase levels in allergic conjunctivitis and vernal keratoconjunctivitis. Cornea. 1994;13(4):345–8. https://doi.org/10.1097/00003226-199407000-00010.
61. Sarac OI, Erdener U, Irkec M, Us D, Gungen Y. Tear eotaxin levels in giant papillary conjunctivitis associated with ocular prosthesis. Ocul Immunol Inflamm. 2003;11(3):223–30. https://doi.org/10.1076/ocii.11.3.223.17350.
62. Zhong X, Liu H, Pu A, Xia X, Zhou X. M cells are involved in pathogenesis of human contact lens-associated giant papillary conjunctivitis. Arch Immunol Ther Exp (Warsz). 2007;55:173–7. https://doi.org/10.1007/s00005-007-0022-x.
63. Korb DR, Allansmith MR, Greiner JV, Henriquez AS, Richmond PP, Finnemore VM. Prevalence of conjunctival changes in wearers of hard contact lenses. Am J Ophthalmol. 1980;90(3):336–41. https://doi.org/10.1016/S0002-9394(14)74913-X.
64. Dumbleton K. Noninflammatory silicone hydrogel contact lens complications. Eye Contact Lens. 2003;29(1):S186–9. https://doi.org/10.1097/00140068-200301001-00051.
65. Takamura E, Uchio E, Ebihara N, Ohno S, Ohashi Y, Okamoto S, Kumagai N, Satake Y, Shoji J, Nakagawa Y, Namba K. Japanese guidelines for allergic conjunctival diseases 2017. Allergol Int. 2017;66(2):220–9. https://doi.org/10.1016/j.alit.2016.12.004.

66. Kymionis GD, Goldman D, Ide T, Yoo SH. Tacrolimus ointment 0.03% in the eye for treatment of giant papillary conjunctivitis. Cornea. 2008;27(2):228–9. https://doi.org/10.1097/ICO.0b013e318159afbb.
67. Lai Y, Sundar G, Ray M. Surgical treatment outcome of medically refractory huge giant papillary conjunctivitis. Am J Ophthalmol Case Rep. 2017;8:22–4. https://doi.org/10.1016/j.ajoc.2017.09.002.

Chapter 4
Infectious Conjunctivitis in Children

Lakshman Mulpuri, Emmanuel Angelo Sarmiento, and Lisa Thompson

Introduction

Background

Conjunctivitis is a common complaint in primary care offices, emergency departments, and eye clinics. The disease can be subdivided into infectious and noninfectious etiologies. This chapter focuses on the various manifestations of infectious conjunctivitis in children to enable the practitioner to recognize the likely source and thus provide timely and appropriate therapeutic options. Acute infectious conjunctivitis is the most common form in the adult population, with viruses responsible for over 80% of cases [1]. Conversely, in the pediatric population, bacteria account for 50–70% of cases [2].

Although overall prognosis is good and rarely leads to vision loss, the economic impact of conjunctivitis is significant. In the United States alone, a study designed to approximate the annual cost of bacterial conjunctivitis estimated an indirect cost ranging from approximately $63 million to $141 million [3]. Infectious conjunctivitis can be highly contagious, with rapid spread in childcare centers and schools. Furthermore, children with infectious conjunctivitis may be absent from school for a significant period of time resulting in increased childcare needs from caretakers

L. Mulpuri
Department of Cornea and External Disease, Bascom Palmer Eye Institute, Miami, FL, USA
e-mail: fi6671@wayne.edu

E. A. Sarmiento · L. Thompson (✉)
Division of Ophthalmology, Cook County Health, Chicago, IL, USA
e-mail: emmanuel.sarmiento@cookcountyhealth.org; lthompson3@cookcountyhhs.org

A. Traish, V. P. Douglas (eds.), *Pediatric Ocular Surface Disease*,
https://doi.org/10.1007/978-3-031-30562-7_4

Table 4.1 Symptoms of conjunctivitis by etiology

Clinical symptoms	Bacterial	Viral	Allergic
Ocular involvement	Bilateral but may be unilateral	Often unilateral but may be bilateral	Bilateral
Discharge	Mucopurulent or sometimes watery	Watery	Watery
Pruritus	Minimal	Minimal	Moderate-severe
Epiphora	Mild-moderate	Severe	Mild-moderate
Lymphadenopathy	Uncommon	Common	None

Notes: Data taken from these sources [4–6]

resulting in potential losses in both economic and social productivity. Therefore it is important to efficiently and accurately diagnose and treat conjunctivitis to facilitate return to school while minimizing the risk of transmission to peers and caregivers.

Some of the most common symptoms of conjunctivitis presentation include, but are not limited to ocular pruritus, redness, discharge, photophobia, tearing, and foreign body sensation. Clinical ambiguity can exist between viral and bacterial presentations since there is some overlap of signs (Table 4.1). Thus, both history-taking and physical examination play a crucial role in differentiating between the etiologies. When examining the bulbar conjunctiva, identifying papillae and follicles can aid in making the diagnosis. Papillae are raised areas of inflammation and edema with central blood vessels; these are more suggestive of a bacterial conjunctivitis. In contrast, follicles are raised lesions that are a collection of plasma cells and lymphocytes without central blood vessels; these are more suggestive of a viral conjunctivitis. Management of infectious conjunctivitis is generally supportive as most cases tend to be self-limited. However, there are various treatment options depending on the etiology.

Risk Factors and Prevention

There are several distinct risk factors which predispose children to both becoming infected and suffering a prolonged course: poor hygiene both with and without contact lens use, a history of ocular surface disease (e.g., dry eye, blepharitis, and lid malposition), a disordered immune system, recent ocular surgery or trauma, and crowded or institutional living [7].

Preventative measures that limit the spread of infection include proper hand hygiene, keeping hands away from the eye, and avoidance of sharing personal items (such as towels) that come in contact with the eyes [7].

Bacterial Conjunctivitis

Overview

There are a number of pathogens known to cause bacterial conjunctivitis. Their incidence in the pediatric population is often correlated with age distributions. After the newborn period, nontypeable *Haemophilus influenzae* is the most common pathogen, accounting for nearly 50–80% of conjunctivitis cases, followed by *Streptococcus pneumoniae* and *Moraxella catarrhalis* [8].

The number of cases attributable to *Streptococcus pneumoniae* varies depending on the patient's age along with their Pneumococcal Conjugate Vaccine (PCV7/13) status. A recent prospective study analyzing the implementation of PCV7/PCV13 vaccines demonstrated significant reductions (93%) in conjunctivitis due to PCV13 serotypes. The study also found reductions in the rates of pneumococcal, nontypeable *Haemophilus influenzae* (NHTi), and overall culture-positive events in children less than 2 years of age [9].

Group A strep pyogenes infections are less common and often occur in school-aged children. *Staphylococcus aureus*, *Neisseria gonorrhoeae*, and *Neisseria meningitidis* are also observed in young children but are exceedingly rare [10].

Presentation

Bacterial conjunctivitis presents with a broad range of symptoms. Unlike its viral counterpart, bacterial conjunctivitis tends to present bilaterally (50–74% of cases) and patients often experience ocular discharge. The discharge is classically purulent but may also be watery and vary in thickness. Conjunctival hyperemia is another common finding and prior studies have demonstrated concurrent hyperemia and discharge as potential indicators of bacterial conjunctivitis [9]. "Gluey" or "sticky" eyelids and physical exam findings of mucoid or purulent discharge were often more predictive of a bacterial etiology [11] (Figs. 4.1 and 4.2). Nonspecific findings in bacterial conjunctivitis include tearing, stinging, light sensitivity, irritation, and/

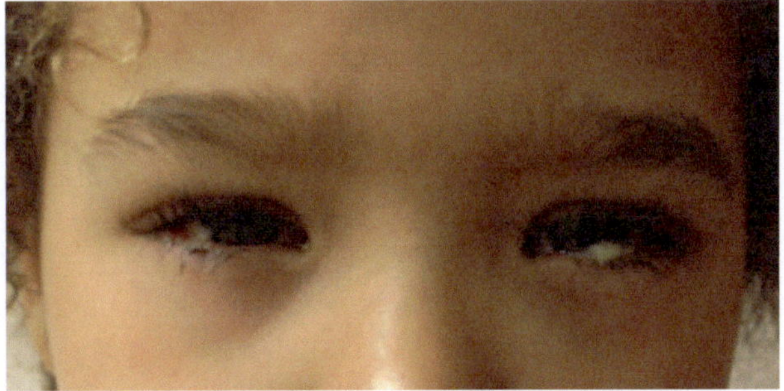

Fig. 4.1 Classic appearance of bacterial conjunctivitis (Courtesy of Lisa Thompson, MD)

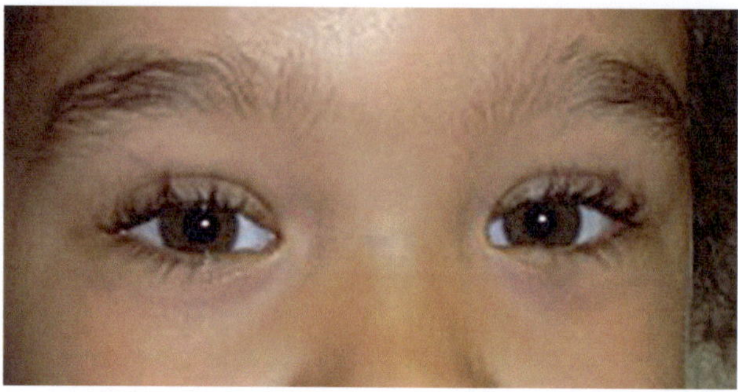

Fig. 4.2 Resolution of bacterial conjunctivitis (Courtesy of Lisa Thompson, MD)

or changes in visual acuity. The incubation period for bacterial pathogens is typically 1 to 3 days [1].

Although most bacterial conjunctivitis cases are self-limited, certain bacterial pathogens possess distinctive clinical features that may aid in diagnosis. *Neisseria gonorrhoeae*, and sometimes *Neisseria meningitidis*, may cause "hyperacute" conjunctivitis, an alarming and rapidly progressive form of conjunctivitis that includes prominent lid edema, excessive and copious purulent discharge along with pseudomembranes, layers of exudative material resembling membranes, and preauricular lymphadenopathy [12].

Chlamydial Conjunctivitis

Chlamydial conjunctivitis is often associated with sexually active teenagers but may present in newborns of infected mothers during delivery. Patients with chlamydia conjunctivitis can also have a concomitant asymptomatic gonococcal infection. It presents in two distinct forms: trachoma and inclusion conjunctivitis. There are over 19 different human serotypes of *Chlamydia trachomatis*. Serotypes D, Da, E, F, G, H, I, Ia, J, and K are associated with inclusion conjunctivitis while serotypes A, B, Ba, and C are usually found in trachoma cases. *Chlamydia trachomatis* is the most common cause of chronic follicular conjunctivitis and is responsible for 20% of acute conjunctivitis cases [4].

In sexually active adolescents, inclusion conjunctivitis often occurs due to poor hygiene and subsequent autoinfection from genital secretions or infection from sexual partners. Patients present with a wide range of symptoms varying in severity. Often, inclusion conjunctivitis presents as a unilateral, chronic follicular conjunctivitis with mucopurulent discharge and is associated with urethritis in men and vaginitis in women [5]. Additional signs and symptoms include preauricular lymphadenopathy, lid swelling, irritation, foreign body sensation, and redness. Without treatment, complications such as peripheral subepithelial corneal infiltrates may occur. Compared to its infectious counterpart, trachoma, inclusion conjunctivitis is self-limited and typically does not lead to blindness.

Repeated infection by Chlamydial serotypes A-C may result in trachoma, a severe, chronic follicular reaction of the superior palpebral conjunctiva. Populations at risk are those with limited environmental and social hygiene resources as well as endemic geographical regions such as parts of North Africa, Middle East, Northwest India, and parts of Southeast Asia. Trachoma affects 400 million individuals worldwide and is the leading cause of preventable blindness [6].

A hallmark finding of trachoma is the presence of follicles on palpebral conjunctiva, seen more prominently on eversion of the upper eyelid. Papillae may form between follicles and coalesce, appearing as thickened and velvety lesions. Additional symptoms during active infection include mucopurulent discharge, papillary hypertrophy, and corneal pannus [13]. Patients may develop a prominent, horizontal band of scar tissue known as Arlt's line. These visible white bands can grow more prominent with repeated insult. Another classic finding in chronic trachoma are Herbert's pits, which are depressions in the upper margin of the cornea due to regression of large follicles [14].

Conjunctival scarring eventually leads to contraction of the palpebral conjunctiva causing cicatricial entropion and trichiasis. Continued insult to the ocular surface from trichiasis leads to profound vision loss due to corneal changes. Scarring, cicatricial entropion and trichiasis, and corneal opacification characterize the final stages of trachoma [6].

Other Bacteria

Bartonella henselae is the most common cause of Parinaud Oculoglandular Syndrome (POGS). This is a unilateral granulomatous follicular conjunctivitis associated with preauricular and submandibular lymphadenopathy. Additional symptoms include serous or mucoid discharge, mild periorbital edema, conjunctival ulceration, and a conjunctival nodule or granuloma. Non-ocular findings include low-grade fever, pain, and suppurative lymphadenopathy. Other causes of POGS in descending order of frequency include *Francisella tularensis*, *Sporothrix schenckii*, *R. typhi/felis* and *R. conorii*, *Mycobacteria tuberculosis*, *Coccidioides immitis*, and *Treponema pallidum* [14].

Diagnosis

The diagnosis of bacterial conjunctivitis is often made clinically. As seen in Table 4.1, unilateral mucopurulent discharge and lack of ocular pruritus are positive predictors of a bacterial etiology. Cultures are indicated for children younger than 2 months, who have severe illnesses or demonstrate copious amounts of discharge. Cultures are also indicated in children who demonstrate resistance to initial empiric therapy, those with a prior history of sexual abuse, or have recurrent conjunctivitis infections [12]. Several organisms may be responsible for bacterial conjunctivitis as seen in Table 4.2 [15].

Table 4.2 Differential diagnosis of bacterial conjunctivitis

Acute and subacute	Chronic	Less common
Neisseria gonorrhea	Staphylococcus aureus	Moraxella catarrhalis
Neisseria meningitides	Moraxella Lacunata	Corynebacterium diphtheriae
Streptococcus pneumoniae		Mycobacterium tuberculosis
Haemophilus influenzae		Chlamydia trachomatis

Note: Data taken from source [15]

Cultures are particularly important in the diagnosis of *Neisseria*, whether it be *Neisseria gonorrhea* (concern for sexual abuse), or *Neisseria meningitidis* (risk for meningitis). Conjunctivitis due to Neisseria requires close follow-up due to concerns of corneal involvement and subsequent vision loss due to the bacteria's lytic enzymes that are able to erode and perforate the eye [16].

When cultures are recommended, conjunctival swabs and two smears for Gram stain and acridine orange should be taken with the swabs cultured on blood and chocolate agar. If chlamydial conjunctivitis is suspected, a conjunctival sample is taken and then run via a monoclonal antibody test that identifies the antigen [17, 18].

Another important consideration when obtaining a history is if the patient is a contact lens wearer. Contact lens use increases the risk of bacterial keratitis, and *Pseudomonas* is the most common infectious organism in this population. Contact lens use should be halted during an infectious conjunctivitis episode [16].

Treatment

Bacterial conjunctivitis tends to resolve spontaneously within 7–10 days. Initial treatment is supportive: warm or cool compresses, artificial tears, frequent hand washing, and avoiding shared items such as towels or cosmetics to prevent spread. Providers can also consider prescribing empiric antibiotics to aid in bacterial clearance and shorten the duration of symptoms to allow for an earlier return to school [7]. In acute non-severe bacterial conjunctivitis: topical aminoglycosides (gentamicin, tobramycin, and neomycin) or fluoroquinolones (ciprofloxacin, ofloxacin, and norfloxacin) can be used in conjunction with bacitracin or erythromycin ointment for a period of 5–7 days.

Admission to the hospital and systemic antibiotic therapy is indicated in more complex scenarios involving immunocompromised patients, such as infants, or suspected cases of *Neisseria gonorrhea* or *Chlamydia* [19]. For *Neisseria gonorrhea*, systemic treatment options include intramuscular ceftriaxone and azithromycin or doxycycline. For *Chlamydia*, systemic treatment options include oral macrolides (azithromycin or erythromycin) and tetracyclines (doxycycline). In advanced cases of trachoma with trichiasis and corneal involvement, surgical correction may be necessary. This may involve redirecting eyelashes and the eyelid margin away from the ocular surface with techniques such as bilateral tarsal rotation or transverse tarsotomy with lid margin rotation [20]. For central corneal scarring, corneal transplantation may be considered to clear the visual axis [20].

Viral Conjunctivitis

Overview

In children, viral conjunctivitis is somewhat less common than its bacterial counterpart. Viruses are transmitted via direct contact with infected fomites, contaminated water, and fecal-oral transmission routes [21]. Nearly 90% of all viral conjunctivitis cases are caused by adenoviruses. In patients younger than 10 years old, adenovirus types 3, 4, 5, and 7 are commonly implicated. Types 8, 19, 37, and 54 are more likely to affect older children and adult populations [1]. Adenoviruses in the pediatric population may manifest as two distinct disease entities: pharyngoconjunctival fever (PCF) or more severe epidemic keratoconjunctivitis (EKC). Herpetic conjunctivitis is another viral infection seen in children. Approximately 1.3–4.8% of acute conjunctivitis cases are caused by the Herpes Simplex Virus (HSV). Finally, picornaviruses EV70 and coxsackievirus A24 variant have been implicated in the development of acute hemorrhagic conjunctivitis, a highly contagious form of viral conjunctivitis [1].

Presentation

Viral conjunctivitis shares many of the symptoms of bacterial conjunctivitis: redness, tearing, photophobia, new foreign body sensation, burning, watery eyes, and discharge. One key distinction is the lack of mucopurulent discharge in viral conjunctivitis. Preauricular lymphadenopathy has a higher association with viral infections but can also be found in more severe bacterial infections such as Neisseria gonorrhoeae. Patients with viral conjunctivitis commonly present with unilateral tearing and follicular injection of the bulbar conjunctiva which commonly spreads to the fellow eye. Incubation time for viral etiologies is longer and with wider variability that ranges between 5 and 14 days [1].

Adenovirus

The most common and least severe ocular manifestation of adenovirus infection in children is conjunctivitis as part of pharyngoconjunctival fever (PCF). It is often caused by types 3, 4, 7 and is characterized by fever, pharyngitis, preauricular lymphadenopathy, and acute follicular conjunctivitis (Fig. 4.3). In addition,

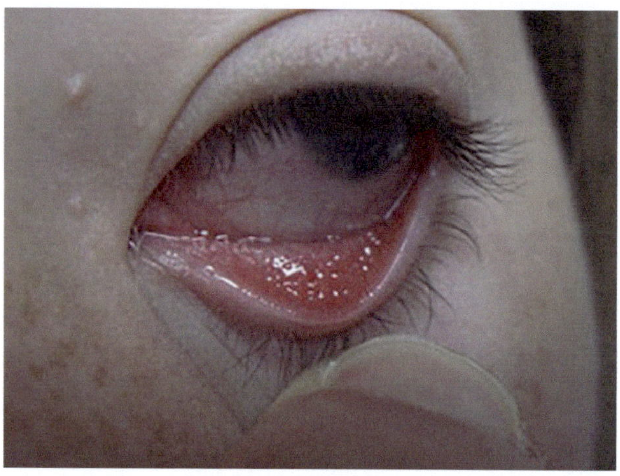

Fig. 4.3 Follicular conjunctivitis (Courtesy of Kenneth W. Wright, MD)

adenovirus replication in the conjunctiva may lead to various ocular findings such as conjunctival hyperemia and edema, and subconjunctival hemorrhage [22]. Fortunately, PCF tends to be a self-limited condition that resolves within 2–3 weeks.

Unlike PCF, Epidemic Keratoconjunctivitis (EKC) is a severe and rapidly progressive form of conjunctivitis due to adenovirus. Unlike PCF, EKC can have a long-lasting impact on the child's visual acuity. In addition to symptoms of redness, tearing, blurry vision, photophobia, and foreign body sensation, patients can present with systemic signs such as generalized malaise, myalgias, and fever. Other ocular manifestations more consistent with EKC include eyelid edema, corneal subepithelial infiltrates, pseudomembranes, and symblepharon [23].

A common sequelae of EKC from adenoviral infection at around 2–4 weeks are subepithelial infiltrates (SEIs). SEIs represent a delayed hypersensitivity response to viral antigens in the corneal stroma and may require topical steroids for a period of weeks to months [23].

Herpes Simplex Virus

A less common viral cause of conjunctivitis is *Herpes Simplex Virus* (HSV). HSV is a double-stranded DNA virus that can reside in the trigeminal ganglion where it stays latent and thus a risk of reactivation can occur [24]. Primary HSV infection occurs through orofacial mucus membrane transmission and usually occurs in children less than 5 years of age. In these children, common features include follicular conjunctivitis, watery discharge, and preauricular lymphadenopathy with characteristic cutaneous vesicular lesions in a dermatomal distribution over the lids with blepharoconjunctivitis. These lesions can continue to spread the virus for up to 10 days and resolve over the course of several weeks [24]. HSV-1 is more often the culprit in the pediatric population [24]. Children compared to older populations are more likely to experience bilateral HSV-1 ocular disease and sequelae of corneal scarring that can be visually significant [24].

In any child with watery discharge and acute follicular conjunctivitis, it is important to consider HSV and culture if appropriate. Herpes simplex ophthalmicus may share a common clinical picture with adenoviral EKC which can lead to misdiagnoses. This challenge was demonstrated by a Japanese study that found 3% of cases diagnosed as EKC by clinical presentation were actually due to HSV [24].

Acute Hemorrhagic Conjunctivitis

Acute Hemorrhagic Conjunctivitis (AHC) is a rare but highly contagious form of conjunctivitis. It is typically caused by enterovirus D70 and coxsackievirus A24 [25]. Patients infected with AHC will experience abrupt onset conjunctival edema, epiphora, eyelid edema, mucus discharge, and subconjunctival hemorrhage (Fig. 4.4). These subconjunctival hemorrhages start as discrete individual hemorrhages but quickly coalesce to become a dramatic red eye [26]. Corneal involvement may include punctate elevations or erosions. Conjunctivitis will clear within 4–6 days but the hemorrhages clear more slowly [27].

Molluscum Contagiosum

Molluscum contagiosum (MC) is an infection caused by a poxvirus and is common in pediatric populations up until 14 years of age. The highest incidence is in children 1–4 years of age. It is transmitted through skin-to-skin contact. Patients will often have a number of small 2–3 mm papular lesions with a classic central depression (umbilication) [28]. Lesions may be found on the lids or on other parts of the child's body. Sometimes the lesion will spontaneously discharge caseous material from the core. Itching, burning, and perilesional erythematous skin are common [29].

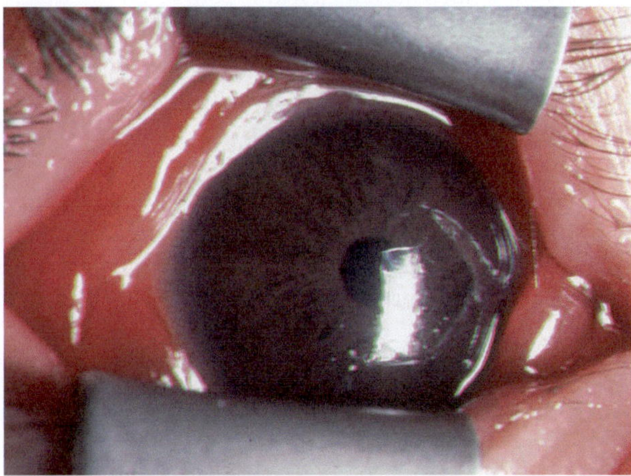

Fig. 4.4 Hemorrhagic conjunctivitis (Courtesy of Kenneth W. Wright, MD)

Lesions involving the margin may shed virus into the conjunctival sac causing unilateral follicular conjunctivitis and less commonly corneal involvement. MC is a self-limited infection that improves within weeks to months without any significant scarring or complications. In immunocompetent individuals, these ocular manifestations will quickly resolve after the skin lesions heal [29].

Diagnosis

In general, the diagnosis of viral conjunctivitis is made clinically. Laboratory testing is rarely indicated unless symptoms persist or infection is prolonged (> 4 weeks). The gold standard for adenoviral testing has been cell culture samples swabbed directly from the conjunctiva. Viral DNA is detected using PCR testing, but this can be costly and time intensive [30].

Treatment

Treatment for adenoviral conjunctivitis is supportive as it is generally self-limited. It consists of symptomatic relief with cold compresses and lubrication with artificial tears. Antihistamine-containing drops have demonstrated efficacy in alleviating ocular pruritic symptoms [31]. If membranes or pseudomembranes are present on slit-lamp examination, they may be removed with Jewelers forceps or an anesthetic soaked cotton swab. Topical antibiotic drops, although not indicated for viral conjunctivitis, are often prescribed [32]. Moreover, topical and oral antiviral therapies demonstrate no benefit in cases of adenoviral conjunctivitis [32].

In cases of herpetic conjunctivitis, topical and/or systemic antiviral therapies are recommended to shorten the course of the disease. Options include topical trifluridine, ganciclovir ophthalmic gel, and oral acyclovir or valacyclovir. Topical corticosteroids should be avoided in herpetic conjunctivitis as they may potentiate the virus. Topical steroid therapy may be indicated in patients with reduced visual acuity due to corneal subepithelial infiltrates upon resolution of the infection [32].

A more recent approach employs povidone-iodine, a common ocular disinfectant, which has demonstrated viability in treating adenoviral conjunctivitis [33]. A single dose in infants with adenoviral conjunctivitis symptoms demonstrated reductions in symptom duration and severity [33].

Neonatal Conjunctivitis

Overview

Neonatal conjunctivitis, also known as ophthalmia neonatorum, usually occurs within the first 4 weeks of life. It is the most common ocular condition in neonates, and infants are typically exposed to infections during delivery [28]. The incidence of infectious neonatal conjunctivitis is between 1 and 2%. Similar to the pediatric population, respiratory bacterial pathogens are implicated in conjunctival causes in newborns. The age of the newborn aids in the discovery of the underlying etiology.

During the first 24 h, chemical conjunctivitis may occur secondary to silver nitrate or from prophylactic drops such as erythromycin or gentamicin. Between 24 and 48 h, bacterial causes of neonatal conjunctivitis such as *Neisseria gonorrhea*, *Staphylococcus aureus*, or exposure to vaginal flora from microbes such as *Escherichia coli, Klebsiella pneumonia, and Staphylococcus epidermidis* should be considered [34]. Between 5 and 14 days, chlamydia trachomatis and herpes kerato-conjunctivitis should be suspected. Infrequently, HSV-2 infection can occur via the birth canal [24]. In addition, *Pseudomonas* can be a causative pathogen for this age group [35].

Presentation

On physical examination, the neonate will commonly present with periorbital edema, conjunctival hyperemia, lid erythema, and purulent discharge. As noted previously, watery discharge is observed in viral etiologies while more purulent discharge is seen in bacterial conjunctivitis. Overall, a less exuberant immune response is seen in neonates due to their immature immune system.

There are unique presentations to each offending organism or agent. Chemical conjunctivitis often presents with mild conjunctival injection and epiphora. *Neisseria gonorrhea* tends to have profuse, purulent discharge along with corneal involvement which may include diffuse epithelial edema and corneal ulceration that may progress to perforation or endophthalmitis if left untreated. Chlamydia has traditional neonatal conjunctival findings in addition to pseudomembranes and may begin with a watery discharge that progresses to a purulent and bloody discharge. Pseudomonas neonatal conjunctivitis often has a green-tinged discharge. Finally, ophthalmia neonatorum secondary to HSV-2 may uniquely present with a periorbital vesicular distribution and corneal involvement in the form of geographic ulceration or dendrites [35].

Diagnosis

A complete physical examination of the neonate is essential. This includes assessing for any systemic symptoms in addition to the ocular presentation. Fluorescein staining can be useful to evaluate for nasolacrimal duct obstruction. A thorough pregnancy history for infectious diseases may enable appropriate consideration of chlamydia and *Neisseria* conjunctivitis. Cultures and Gram stain assessment of neonatal discharge may be critical when considering certain pathogens since some populations are at higher risk. For example, infants born to HIV-positive mothers have higher incidences of neonatal conjunctivitis [36].

Treatment

After determining the etiology of the neonate's conjunctivitis, various therapies are indicated. Chemical conjunctivitis often resolves within 2–4 days. The most common cause of conjunctivitis, *Chlamydia trachomatis*, is treated with topical and oral erythromycin for a period of 2–3 weeks. Topical formulations alone are less efficacious due to chlamydia's colonization of the nasopharynx and subsequent spread to the lungs if inadequately treated. Thus these neonates should also be assessed for systemic signs of chlamydial infection. Neonates given systemic erythromycin therapy should be closely followed to manage the risks of pyloric stenosis associated with macrolides [37].

Gonococcal conjunctivitis is considered a serious medical emergency and warrants immediate pharmacologic intervention. Third-generation cephalosporins such as ceftriaxone are commonly utilized. If there are signs of disseminated infection, a prolonged course of antibiotics between 7 and 14 days is necessary. Additionally, erythromycin or bacitracin ophthalmic ointment should be applied to the neonate's eyes every 2–4 h and mucopurulent discharge should be irrigated every 1–2 h with normal saline. Neonates with gonococcal conjunctivitis should also be treated for chlamydia due to the high rate of concomitant infection [37].

Neonates with herpetic conjunctivitis may be treated with topical vidarabine or trifluridine 5–6 times daily in addition to oral acyclovir for 14–21 days. These infants should be assessed for systemic signs of herpes infection. In addition, mothers and partners should be counseled and treated [37].

Conclusion

Infectious conjunctivitis is a common and highly contagious pediatric ocular disease with variable clinical presentation. In this chapter, the causative pathogens are presented along with the clinical features, diagnostic approach, and treatment options. Understanding the different pathogens and their varying clinical presentations is crucial for initiation of proper management for this unique population.

References

1. Azari AA, Barney NP. Conjunctivitis. JAMA. 2013;310(16):1721.
2. Taddio A, Cimaz R, Caputo R, de Libero C, Di Grande L, Simonini G, et al. Childhood chronic anterior uveitis associated with vernal keratoconjunctivitis (VKC): successful treatment with topical tacrolimus. Case series. Pediatr Rheumatol. 2011;9(1):34.
3. Smith AF, Waycaster C. Estimate of the direct and indirect annual cost of bacterial conjunctivitis in the United States. BMC Ophthalmol. 2009;9(1)
4. Fitch CP, Rapoza PA, Owens S, Murillo-Lopez F, Johnson RA, Quinn TC, et al. Epidemiology and diagnosis of acute conjunctivitis at an inner-city hospital. Ophthalmology. 1989;96(8):1215–20.
5. Darville T. Chlamydia trachomatis infections in neonates and young children. Semin Pediatr Infect Dis. 2005;16(4):235–44.
6. Ahmad B, Patel BC. Trachoma. In: StatPearls [internet]. Treasure Island, FL: StatPearls Publishing; 2022.
7. Azari AA, Arabi A. Conjunctivitis: A systematic review. J Ophthalmic Vis Res. 2020;15(3):372–95.
8. Leung AKC, Hon KL, Wong AHC, Wong AS. Bacterial conjunctivitis in childhood: etiology, clinical manifestations, diagnosis, and management. Recent Patents Inflamm Allergy Drug Discov. 2018;12(2):120–7.
9. Dagan R, Ben-Shimol S, Greenberg D, Givon-Lavi N. A prospective, population-based study to determine the incidence and bacteriology of bacterial conjunctivitis in children <2 years of age following 7-valent and 13-valent pneumococcal conjugate vaccine sequential implementation. Clin Infect Dis. 2020;72(7):1200–7.
10. Block S. Pediatric acute bacterial conjunctivitis: An update [Internet]. Healio. 2011; [cited 2022Aug1]. https://www.healio.com/news/pediatrics/20120331/pediatric-acute-bacterial-conjunctivitis-an-update
11. Patel PB, Diaz MC, Bennett JE, Attia MW. Clinical features of bacterial conjunctivitis in children. Acad Emerg Med. 2007;14(1):1–5.
12. Chawla R, Kellner JD, Astle WF. Acute infectious conjunctivitis in childhood. Paediatr Child Health. 2001;6(6):329–35.
13. Keenan JD, Lietman TM. Chlamydial infections. In: Cornea. 4th ed. Elsevier Mosby; 2016. p. 503–7.
14. Dixon MK, Dayton CL, Anstead GM. Parinaud's OCULOGLANDULAR syndrome: A case in an adult with flea-borne typhus and a review. Trop Med Infect Dis. 2020;5(3):126.
15. Yeu E, Hauswirth S. A review of the differential diagnosis of acute infectious conjunctivitis: implications for treatment and management. Clin Ophthalmol. 2020;14:805–13.
16. Donahue SP, Khoury JM, Kowalski RP. Common ocular infections. Drugs. 1996;52(4):526–40.
17. Byrne KA. Diagnostic microbiology and cytology of the eye. J Clin Pathol. 1996;49(9):780.
18. Seal DV, Pleyer U. Ocular infection. New York: Informa Healthcare USA; 2007.
19. Pippin MM, Le JK. Bacterial Conjunctivitis. In: StatPearls [Internet]. Treasure Island, FL: StatPearls Publishing; 2022.
20. Rajak SN, Collin JR, Burton MJ. Trachomatous trichiasis and its management in endemic countries. Surv Ophthalmol. 2012;57(2):105–35.
21. Solano D, Fu L, Czyz CN. Viral Conjunctivitis. In: StatPearls [Internet]. Treasure Island, FL: StatPearls Publishing; 2022.
22. Chigbu DG, Labib B. Pathogenesis and management of adenoviral keratoconjunctivitis. Infect Drug Resist. 2018;11:981–93.

23. Pihos AM. Epidemic keratoconjunctivitis: A review of current concepts in management. J Opt. 2013;6(2):69–74.
24. Kanukollu VM, Patel BC. Herpes simplex ophthalmicus. In: StatPearls [Internet]. Treasure Island, FL: StatPearls Publishing; 2022.
25. Mescar K, Modlin J, Abzug M. Enteroviruses and Parechoviruses. In: Principles and practice of pediatric infectious disease, fifth. Philadelphia, PA: Elsevier; 2018. p. 1205–13.
26. Khan A, Sharif S, Shaukat S, Khan S, Zaidi S. An outbreak of acute hemorrhagic conjunctivitis (AHC) caused by coxsackievirus A24 variant in Pakistan. Virus Res. 2008;137(1):150–2.
27. Wairagkar NS. Acute hemorrhagic conjunctivitis 077.4 (epidemic hemorrhagic conjunctivitis, apollo 11 disease). In: Roy FH, Fraunfelder FW, Fraunfelder FT, Tindall R, Jensvold B, editors. Roy and Fraunfelder's current ocular therapy. Pune: Elsevier; 2008. p. 10–1.
28. Makker K, Nassar G, Kaufman E. Neonatal conjunctivitis. In: StatPearls [Internet]. Treasure Island, FL: StatPearls Publishing; 2022.
29. Meza-Romero R, Navarrete-Dechent C, Downey C. Molluscum contagiosum: an update and review of new perspectives in etiology, diagnosis, and treatment. Clin Cosmet Investig Dermatol. 2019;12:373–81.
30. Usman N, Suarez M. Adenoviruses. In: StatPearls [Internet]. Treasure Island, FL: StatPearls Publishing; 2022.
31. Varu DM, Rhee MK, Akpek EK, Amescua G, Farid M, Garcia-Ferrer FJ, et al. Conjunctivitis preferred practice pattern®. Ophthalmology. 2019;126(1):P94–P169.
32. Shekhawat NS, Shtein RM, Blachley TS, Stein JD. Antibiotic prescription fills for acute conjunctivitis among enrollees in a large United States managed care network. Ophthalmology. 2017;124(8):1099–107.
33. Özen Tunay Z, Ozdemir O, Petricli IS. Povidone iodine in the treatment of adenoviral conjunctivitis in infants. Cutan Ocul Toxicol. 2014;34(1):12–5.
34. Kara M, Kıvanç SA, Olcaysü OO, Akova Budak B, Özmen AT, Kıvanç M, et al. The newborn conjunctival flora at the post delivery 24 hours. J Curr Ophthalmol. 2018;30(4):348–52.
35. Mehner LC, Singh JK. Ocular disorders in the newborn. NeoReviews. 2021;22:7.
36. Mahon BE, Rosenman MB, Kleiman MB. Maternal and infant use of erythromycin and other macrolide antibiotics as risk factors for infantile hypertrophic pyloric stenosis. J Pediatr. 2001;139(3):380–4.
37. Zikic A, Schünemann H, Wi T, Lincetto O, Broutet N, Santesso N. Treatment of neonatal chlamydial conjunctivitis: A systematic review and meta-analysis. J Pediatr Infect Dis Soc. 2018;7(3):e107–15.

Chapter 5
Ocular Surface Lesions in Children

Leyla Yavuz Saricay, Prashant Yadav, Anna M. Stagner,
and Jenny C. Dohlman

Introduction

A variety of ocular surface lesions can occur in children and can be categorized as choristomatous, epithelial, melanocytic, vascular, fibrous, xanthomatous, or lymphoid, among others [1–4]. In a clinical series of 262 children with a conjunctival tumor, most were of melanocytic origin (67%), choristomas (10%), and vascular tumors or malformations (9%) followed in frequency [1]. The clinical presentation of these lesions is varied with regard to localization (corneal, limbal, conjunctival, bulbar), origin (malformation or neoplasia), character (solid, cystic), histopathology (benign, malignant, inflammatory/reactive), and age of presentation (congenital or acquired) as compared to similar tumors in adults [5].

While the majority of ocular surface tumors in children are benign, in this population, they may impact vision and result in significant morbidity [1–3, 6], making diagnostic accuracy crucial in the pediatric population due to the risk of amblyopia. Permanent vision loss may occur from obscuration of the visual axis or induced corneal astigmatism [1, 2, 5, 7]. The diagnosis of pediatric ocular surface tumors is usually made on a clinical basis, taking into account age of presentation, history of growth, and the localization or pattern of the lesion [2]. An incisional biopsy is

L. Y. Saricay · J. C. Dohlman (✉)
Department of Ophthalmology, Boston Children's Hospital, Harvard Medical School,
Boston, MA, USA
e-mail: Leyla.YavuzSaricay@childrens.harvard.edu; Jenny.dohlman@childrens.harvard.edu

P. Yadav · A. M. Stagner
Massachusetts Eye and Ear Infirmary, Department of Ophthalmology, Harvard Medical
School, Boston, MA, USA
e-mail: Prashant_yadav2@meei.harvard.edu; Anna_stagner@meei.harvard.edu

A. Traish, V. P. Douglas (eds.), *Pediatric Ocular Surface Disease*,
https://doi.org/10.1007/978-3-031-30562-7_5

occasionally performed when the lesion cannot be diagnosed clinically; excisional biopsy may be needed for prevention of amblyopia [4].

Herein, we review the benign and malignant ocular surface neoplasms and malformations and discuss their common clinical presentations and histopathologic findings, along with diagnostic approaches and management strategies.

Epithelial-Derived Conjunctival Tumors

Pterygium

Pterygium is a very common disorder of the ocular surface which presents with a triangular or wing-shaped encroachment of abnormal bulbar conjunctival tissue onto the cornea [8]. Etiology is likely multifactorial and may involve certain geographic locations and climates, excessive and prolonged sunlight exposure, and ultraviolet (UV) radiation [9]. Surgical intervention may be considered for pediatric patients when there is persistent discomfort, chronic irritation, recurrent inflammation, visual distortion or amblyopia risk in the setting of irregular astigmatism, restricted ocular motility, or poor cosmesis [10]. Out of all techniques, conjunctival autografting is the best available option after pterygium excision to prevent recurrence [9, 10]. Histopathology shows subepithelial fibrosis with vascular ectasia and varying amounts of solar elastosis and reactive epithelial changes.

Epithelial Inclusion Cyst

Conjunctival inclusion cysts are benign and non-neoplastic and may present primarily or secondarily. Primary conjunctival inclusion cysts are present at birth and increase in size over time. The most common location is the superior nasal bulbar conjunctiva which can often involve the limbus. These lesions can progress to involve the cornea and can result in amblyopia. Secondary conjunctival inclusion cysts are more commonly caused by trauma, ocular surgery, or chronic inflammation resulting in the separation of the conjunctival epithelium [11].

Patients are generally asymptomatic, but larger conjunctival inclusion cysts can affect vision and cause a foreign body sensation or eye pain. The diagnosis of conjunctival inclusion cysts is mostly clinical, and the histopathologic examination of excised cysts shows a non-keratinized stratified squamous mucosal lining with varying amount of goblet cells and serous or mucinous, acellular content. The differential diagnosis of pinguecula/pterygium, nodular scleritis, conjunctival lymphangiectasia, and phlyctenule may be considered when evaluating cystic masses of the conjunctiva [11, 12].

Papilloma

Conjunctival papilloma is a benign tumor that is usually associated with low-risk human papillomavirus, especially types 6 and 11 [13]. It is speculated that the virus is acquired as the child passes through the mother's birth canal. Papillomas appear as pink to red, filiform epithelial proliferations with fibrovascular cores [13]. In childhood, papillomas represent 7% to 10% of conjunctival tumors [14]. Conjunctival papillomas may be sessile or pedunculated, with a typical "cauliflower -like" appearance. The most common presentation is within the inferior fornix or at the limbus. Small lesions may be observed because of their high rate of spontaneous resolution [1, 4, 5, 14].

Ocular Surface Squamous Neoplasia

Ocular surface squamous neoplasia is uncommon in children and is usually secondary to immunosuppressive conditions like human immunodeficiency virus, underlying DNA repair abnormalities such as xeroderma pigmentosum, or organ transplantation [15]. Histopathologically, conjunctival intraepithelial neoplasia (CIN) shows atypical squamous cells that do not span the full thickness of the epithelium; squamous cell carcinoma results when the dysplastic cells extend through the basement membrane into the conjunctival substantia propria [15]. Clinically, invasive squamous cell carcinoma tends to be larger and more elevated than CIN. Leukoplakia may be seen in both conditions. The management of the ocular surface malignancies can include topical medical therapies and/or surgical excision with cryotherapy [15].

Melanocytic Conjunctival Tumors

Nevus

Conjunctival nevi are the most common melanocytic tumors in childhood; they may be congenital or acquired, but may not become clinically apparent until adolescence. Conjunctival nevi can manifest as darkly pigmented (65%), lightly pigmented (19%), or completely amelanotic (16%) [1, 16–18]. They are typically located within the interpalpebral bulbar conjunctiva near the limbus and usually remain stationary throughout life, although growth may occur during puberty. Nevi are very often cystic and should move freely with the conjunctiva. Management is conservative because the malignant transformation of conjunctival nevi is extremely rare in childhood (<1%) [1, 2, 4, 16, 18–20]. Histopathologically, nevi are well-nested, with banal appearing melanocytes within the epithelium and substantia

Fig. 5.1 Compound nevus

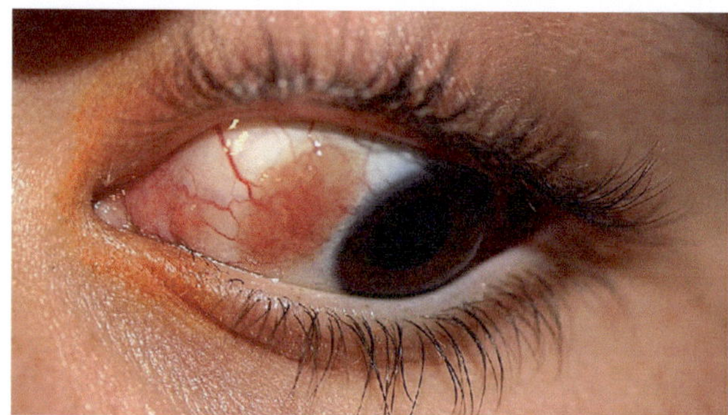

Fig. 5.2 A 9-year-old with a pigmented lesion of the bulbar conjunctiva, hematoxylin, and eosin, 20x. This compound nevus shows junctional melanocytic nests with the epithelium as well as within the substantia propria. There are associated epithelial inclusion cysts, typically a feature of benignity

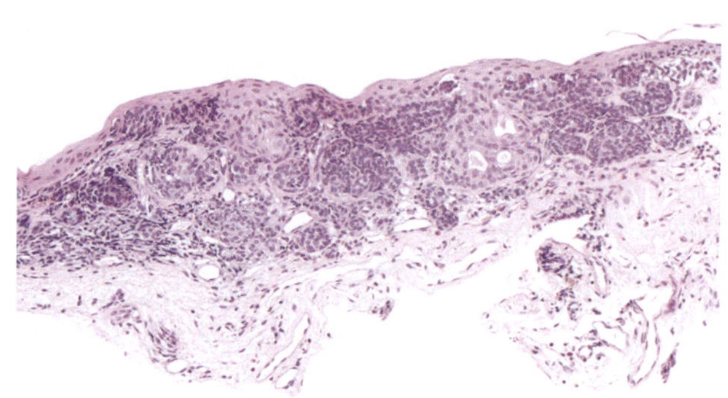

propria. Like cutaneous nevi, they may be junctional, compound (Figs. 5.1 and 5.2), or subepithelial, and may show an associated inflammatory infiltrate. Like in skin, a robust junctional component is often present. The management is usually observation [1, 16, 18–20].

Ocular Melanocytosis

Ocular melanocytosis is characterized by congenital hyperpigmentation of the episclera, resulting in slate-gray colored, discrete patches underneath the conjunctiva. Typically, there is no intraepithelial conjunctival pigment [1]. Therefore, unlike conjunctival nevi, episcleral melanosis does not move with the overlying conjunctiva. It is more commonly seen in darkly pigmented individuals. If it is accompanied by hyperpigmentation of the eyelid, the term nevus of Ota is applied [1]. Scleral involvement occurs in greater than two-thirds of cases and is associated with an increased risk of developing glaucoma [21]. Nevus of Ota is typically benign with an excellent ophthalmic and dermatologic prognosis with or without treatment.

Yearly screening for glaucoma and malignant melanoma by an ophthalmologist and dermatologist is recommended [21]. This condition imparts a 1 in 400 risk for the development of uveal melanoma, as the melanocytes are dendritic and deep, but there is no increased risk of conjunctival melanoma. Affected patients should be followed once or twice yearly for the development of uveal, orbital, or meningeal melanoma [1, 6, 16, 18].

Vascular Conjunctival Tumors

Capillary (Infantile) Hemangioma

Hemangiomas are benign tumors, and in this age group typically fall into the capillary category. Infantile hemangioma presents in infancy as a reddish stromal mass, sometimes associated with a cutaneous orbital component, with a rapid growth phase in the subsequent 6 months (Fig. 5.3) [1, 17]. Similar to cutaneous infantile hemangiomas, the conjunctival hemangioma enlarges over several months and then spontaneously involutes. Most commonly, the management of conjunctival capillary hemangiomas is observation, but surgical resection or local or systemic propranolol or prednisone may be needed [1, 5, 14, 17].

Lymphangioma

The ocular surface lymphangioma is a slowly progressive vascular malformation of lymphatic or venolymphatic channels which may present as an isolated conjunctival lesion or can be a component of a deeper diffuse orbital lymphangioma [1, 5, 17, 18]. It usually becomes clinically apparent in the first decade of life, with

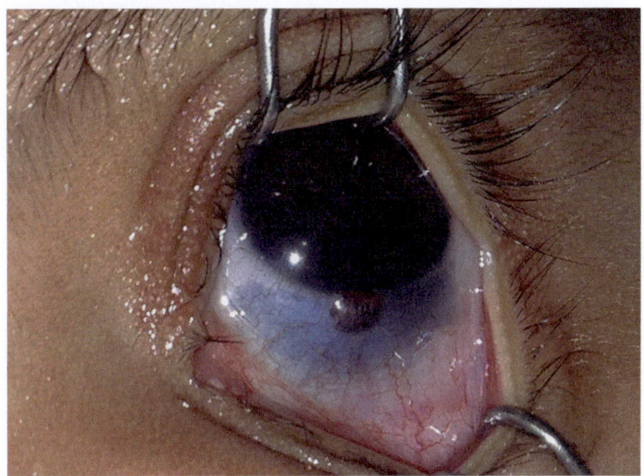

Fig. 5.3 Capillary hemangioma

variable-sized clear dilated cystic channels. Unlike infantile hemangioma, it does not involute. In some cases, blood is visible in many of the cystic lesions, giving it the name "chocolate cysts" [22]. The treatment of conjunctival lymphangioma is often difficult because surgical resection or radiotherapy cannot completely eradicate the mass [1].

Pyogenic Granuloma

Pyogenic granulomas in the context of ophthalmology are described as benign, non-neoplastic vascular tumors which are considered a proliferative fibrovascular response to prior tissue insult by chronic inflammation, surgery, chalazion, or non-surgical trauma [1, 5, 14, 16]. Pyogenic granulomas present as red, beefy, pedunculated masses that grow rapidly and consist of fibroblasts and capillaries (Fig. 5.4). Histologically, they are composed of granulation tissue with acute and chronic inflammatory cells and numerous small-caliber blood vessels comprised of plump endothelial cells (Fig. 5.5). Neither suppurative nor granulomatous, the term "pyogenic granuloma" is a a misnomer. Lobular capillary hemangioma, which is a synonym for pyogenic granuloma at other tissue sites, is felt to be a true neoplasm. Treatment includes topical steroids or excision of the lesion [1].

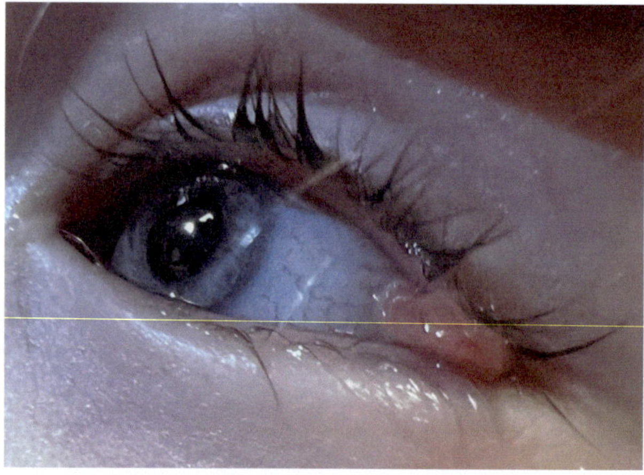

Fig. 5.4 Pyogenic granuloma

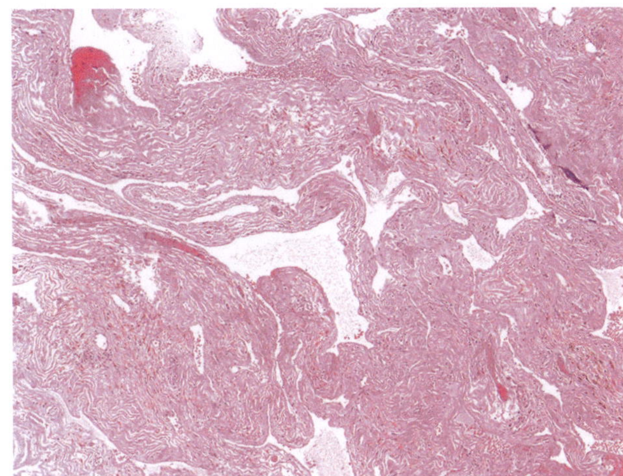

Fig. 5.5 A 16-year-old with an orbital "lymphangioma," hematoxylin, and eosin, 10x. Orbital lymphangiomas are technically venolymphatic malformations comprised of anastomosing thin-walled vessels containing blood (top) and lymph (bottom). There is hemosiderin depositional within the walls, consistent with prior hemorrhage in this lesion

Choristomatous Tumors

A choristoma is a developmental mass-like growth of histologically normal tissue in an abnormal location. Ocular choristomas can be classified as dermoid, dermolipoma, complex choristoma (choristomas with more than one tissue type), and single-tissue choristomas [1, 2, 4].

Dermoid

Dermoid tumors (in contrast to dermoid cysts), the most common type of episcleral choristomas in children, are congenital well-circumscribed, yellow-white solid masses involving the surface of the globe (Fig. 5.6) [23]. The tumors can be unilateral or bilateral and are primarily located in regions of the bulbar conjunctiva (usually inferotemporal quadrant), limbus, cornea, and/or caruncles [23]. Limbal dermoids consist of stratified squamous epithelium with underlying dense dermal-type collagen and associated adnexal structures (Fig. 5.7) and have been classified into three grades clinically [3, 4, 11, 14, 24–26]. Grade I describes superficial lesions less than 5 mm in the limbal area, which may create anisometropic amblyopia by flattening the cornea next to the lesion. Grade II refers to larger lesions

Fig. 5.6 Limbal dermoid

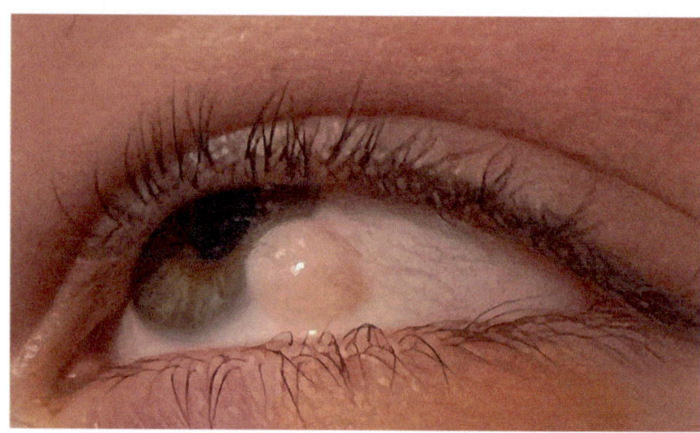

Fig. 5.7 A 2-year-old with a solid limbal dermoid, hematoxylin, and eosin, 10x. Beneath the conjunctival epithelium, the substantia propria is replaced by dense dermis-like collagen containing folliculosebaceous units and lobules of adipose tissue

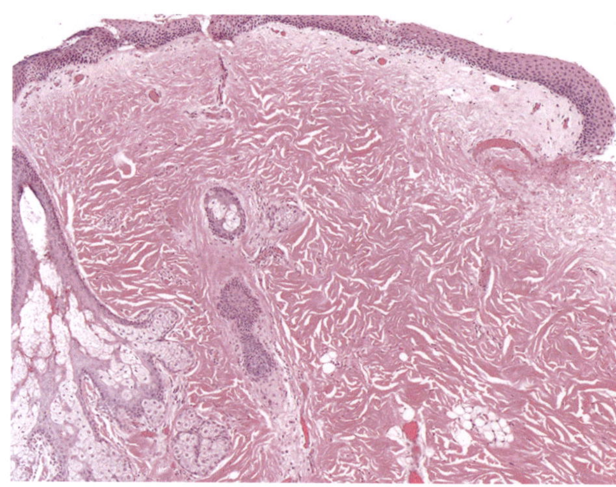

located in both the cornea and limbal area, which may extend to stroma and Descemet's membrane. Grade III describes larger tumors that may spread to other anterior segment structures such as the iris [3, 27].

Limbal dermoids are congenital and may increase in size [28]. They may rarely be associated with Goldenhar's syndrome, which is characterized by a triad of anomalies including epibulbar dermoids, accessory auricular appendages, and aural fistulas. It may also be associated with vertebral, cardiac, renal, and central nervous system defects [7, 29–32]. The management of dermoids that are small and not causing vision-threatening sequelae is observation. Nevertheless, it is recommended that these children undergo close clinical observation with serial examinations in the office, not only to monitor stability but to ensure proper visual development and to provide reassurance for parents [6, 23].

Dermolipoma

Dermolipomas are asymptomatic, benign, congenital solid masses that are typically found along the temporal aspect of the globe and might not be detected until adulthood [2, 4, 5, 16, 28, 33, 34]. They present as soft, fluctuant masses with fine white hairs on their surface [9, 24]. Dermolipomas tend to be unilateral and generally do not interfere with vision due to their superotemporal localization [27, 33–37]. Similar to dermoids, they can be associated with Goldenhar's syndrome [29–32]. Dermolipomas have features similar to orbital fat on computed tomography (CT) and magnetic resonance imaging (MRI) [38]. They consist of dense collagenous and adipose tissue lined by stratified squamous epithelium, typically occurring in the superotemporal conjunctival fornix [1, 2, 4, 17, 34, 35]. The majority of dermolipomas require no treatment, but surgical debulking can be performed for enlarging lesions or lesions causing surface irritation, without necessarily aiming for complete excision [35, 38–42]. In adults, there is significant clinical and histopathologic overlap with prolapsed orbital fat.

Epibulbar Osseous Choristoma

Epibulbar osseous choristoma, composed of mature cortical bone, is the rarest type of choristoma of the ocular surface in the pediatric population. Osseous choristomas are usually found in the superotemporal quadrant (Fig. 5.8) and demonstrate a calcium component on ultrasonography or CT. It is reported that epibulbar osseous choristomas have limited to no growth potential; however, periodic follow-up is still recommended [1, 2, 17].

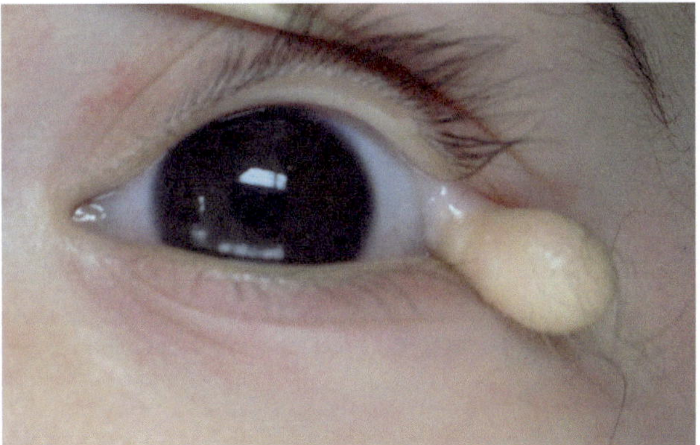

Fig. 5.8 Epibulbar osseous choristoma

Complex Choristoma

Complex choristoma is the rarest type of choristoma with more than two normal tissues growing in an abnormal location. Complex choristoma may be sporadic or associated with systemic diseases, such as nevus sebaceous disease, which includes cutaneous and neurologic features. Cartilage, accessory lacrimal gland, smooth and skeletal muscle, and adipose tissue are common composite elements [1, 2, 5, 7, 17].

Conclusion

Most ocular surface tumors of childhood are benign congenital tumors that are distinct from tumors that occur in adults. Rarely, ocular surface tumors in childhood are malignant or undergo malignant transformation. The majority of pediatric ocular surface tumors are pigmented or non-pigmented nevi with prominent intralesional cysts and rarely evolve into melanoma (<1%). Episcleral melanocytosis may be a sign of possible uveal melanocytosis, so children with this condition should be dilated once or twice a year, as there is a small risk for the development of uveal melanoma. Whereas malignant tumors may be life-threatening, both malignant and benign tumors may be vision-threatening, so amblyopia risk and monitoring for proper visual development are also essential during the follow-up for children with ocular surface lesions.

References

1. Shields CL, Shields JA. Conjunctival tumors in children. Curr Opin Ophthalmol. 2007;18:351–60.
2. Shields CL, Sioufi K, Alset AE, et al. Clinical features differentiating benign from malignant conjunctival tumors in children. JAMA Ophthalmol. 2017;135:215–24.
3. Shields JA, Kaden IH, Eagle RC, et al. Orbital dermoid cysts: clinicopathologic correlations, classification, and management. The 1997 Josephine E. Schueler Lecture. Ophthalmic Plast Reconstr Surg. 1997, 13:265–76.
4. Zimmermann-Paiz MA, García de la Riva JC. Conjunctival tumors in children: histopathologic diagnosis in 165 cases. Arq Bras Oftalmol. 2015;78:337–9.
5. Castillo BV, Kaufman L. Pediatric tumors of the eye and orbit. Pediatr Clin N Am. 2003;50:149–72.
6. Singh AD, De Potter P, Fijal BA, et al. Lifetime prevalence of uveal melanoma in white patients with oculo(dermal) melanocytosis. Ophthalmology. 1998;105:195–8.
7. Rao AA, Naheedy JH, Chen JY-Y, et al. A clinical update and radiologic review of pediatric orbital and ocular tumors. J Oncol. 2013;2013:975908.
8. Panchapakesan J, Hourihan F, Mitchell P. Prevalence of pterygium and pinguecula: the Blue Mountains eye study. Aust N Z J Ophthalmol. 1998;26(Suppl 1):S2–5.

9. Yadav AR, Bhattad KR, Sen PA, et al. Outcome of different techniques of pterygium excision with conjunctival autografting in pediatric population: our experience in central India. Indian J Ophthalmol. 2015;63:491–5.
10. Detorakis ET, Spandidos DA. Pathogenetic mechanisms and treatment options for ophthalmic pterygium: trends and perspectives (review). Int J Mol Med. 2009;23:439–47.
11. Thatte S, Jain J, Kinger M, et al. Clinical study of histologically proven conjunctival cysts. Saudi J Ophthalmol. 2015;29:109–15.
12. Imaizumi M, Nagata M, Matsumoto CS, et al. Primary conjunctival epithelial cyst of the orbit. Int Ophthalmol. 2007;27:269–71.
13. Scott IU, Karp CL, Nuovo GJ. Human papillomavirus 16 and 18 expression in conjunctival intraepithelial neoplasia. Ophthalmology. 2002;109:542–7.
14. Elsas FJ, Green WR. Epibulbar tumors in childhood. Am J Ophthalmol. 1975;79:1001–7.
15. Höllhumer R, Williams S, Michelow P. Ocular surface squamous neoplasia: management and outcomes. Eye (Lond). 2021;35:1562–73.
16. Shields CL, Shields JA. Tumors of the conjunctiva and cornea. Surv Ophthalmol. 2004;49:3–24.
17. Shields CL, Shields JA. Tumors of the conjunctiva and cornea. Indian J Ophthalmol. 2019;67:1930–48.
18. Spraul CW, Grossniklaus HE. Tumors of the cornea and conjunctiva. Curr Opin Ophthalmol. 1996;7:28–34.
19. Heffler KF. Tumors of the cornea and conjunctiva. Curr Opin Ophthalmol. 1995;6:32–8.
20. Ciuntu RE, Martinescu G, Anton N, et al. Conjunctival melanocytic tumors in children - a challenge in diagnosis and treatment. Romanian J Morphol Embryol. 2018;59:317–22.
21. Hori Y, Takayama O. Circumscribed dermal melanoses. Classification and histologic features. Dermatol Clin. 1988;6:315–26.
22. Eiferman RA, Gushard RH. Chocolate cysts of the orbit. Ann Ophthalmol. 1986;18:156–7.
23. Pirouzian A. Management of pediatric corneal limbal dermoids. Clin Ophthalmol. 2013;7:607–14.
24. Bonavolontà G, Tranfa F, de Conciliis C, et al. Dermoid cysts: 16-year survey. Ophthalmic Plast Reconstr Surg. 1995;11:187–92.
25. Eldrup-Forgensen P. Primary, histologically confirmed orbital tumours in Denmark 1943-1962. Histopathological and prognostic studies. Acta Ophthalmol (Copenh). 1970;48:657–66.
26. Shields JA, Shields CL. Orbital cysts of childhood—classification, clinical features, and management. Surv Ophthalmol. 2004;49:281–99.
27. Kamali K, El-Rifai null. Dermolipoma adherent to the lacrimal gland. Bull Ophthalmol Soc Egypt. 1975;68:633–6.
28. Wilde C, Vahdani K, Thaung C, et al. Presenting features for developmental cysts of the orbit. Eye (Lond). 2023;37(2):309–12. https://doi.org/10.1038/s41433-022-01929-3.
29. Berkman MD, Feingold M. Oculoauriculovertebral dysplasia (Goldenhar's syndrome). Oral Surg Oral Med Oral Pathol. 1968;25:408–17.
30. Nkrumah FK. Oculoauriculovertebral dysplasia (Goldenhar's syndrome). Ghana Med J. 1971;10:60–2.
31. Solovjev M. Oculoauriculovertebral dysplasia (Goldenhar's syndrome) (author's transl). Radiol Diagn (Berl). 1978;19:70–5.
32. Mansour AM, Wang F, Henkind P, et al. Ocular findings in the facioauriculovertebral sequence (Goldenhar-Gorlin syndrome). Am J Ophthalmol. 1985;100:555–9.
33. Garg N, Panikar N. Epibulbar dermolipoma. Indian J Pathol Microbiol. 2013;56:477–8.
34. Guimaraes W. Desmoid tumors: lipoma and subconjunctival dermolipoma, general considerations and case presentations. Rev Bras Oftalmol. 1956;15:55–61.
35. Beby F, Kodjikian L, Roche O, et al. Conjunctival tumors in children. A histopathologic study of 42 cases. J Fr Ophtalmol. 2005;28:817–23.
36. Cernea P, Vasile L. Epibulbar dermolipoma. Rev Chir Oncol Radiol O R L Oftalmol Stomatol Ser Oftalmol. 1987;31:211–4.

37. Consul BN, Charan H, Sharma DP. Ocular dermolipoma with congenital mesodermal deformities. J Indian Med Assoc. 1968;51:349–50.
38. Kim E, Kim H-J, Kim Y-D, et al. Subconjunctival fat prolapse and dermolipoma of the orbit: differentiation on CT and MR imaging. AJNR Am J Neuroradiol. 2011;32:465–7.
39. Fry CL, Leone CR. Safe management of dermolipomas. Arch Ophthalmol. 1994;112:1114–6.
40. McNab AA, Wright JE, Caswell AG. Clinical features and surgical management of dermolipomas. Aust N Z J Ophthalmol. 1990;18:159–62.
41. Sa H-S, Kim HK, Shin JH, et al. Dermolipoma surgery with rotational conjunctival flaps. Acta Ophthalmol. 2012;90:86–90.
42. Vahdani K, Rose GE. The presentation and surgical treatment of peribulbar dermolipomas. Ophthalmic Plast Reconstr Surg. 2021;37:226–9.

Chapter 6
Pediatric Ocular Graft-Versus-Host Disease and Dry Eye Disease

Manokamna Agarwal, Simon S. M. Fung, Kamiar Mireskandari, and Asim Ali

Hematopoietic Stem Cell Transplantation (HSCT)

Hematopoietic stem cell transplantation (HSCT) is a highly specialized form of immune therapy that re-establishes blood cell production in patients with acute and chronic leukemia, lymphoma, multiple myeloma, inherited disorders like severe combined immunodeficiency and thalassemia, and other inborn errors of metabolism [1]. Depending on the source of the hematopoietic cells, the HSCT can be *autologous*, involving transplantation of hematopoietic stem cells (HSCs) from the patient's own bone marrow and re-infusion after high doses of cytotoxic therapy; *allogeneic*, involving transfusion of multipotent HSCs in bone marrow, peripheral blood, or umbilical cord blood from a healthy donor who is typically human leukocyte antigen (HLA) matched; and *syngeneic*, when the healthy donor is an identical twin of the patient [2]. From 1957 to 2016, over 1.2 million HSCTs have been performed with 57% being autologous. The global rate of HSCT is approximately 84,000/year [3]. The rate of HSCT has increased over the years. Data in 2016

M. Agarwal
Department of Ophthalmology and Vision Sciences, Hospital for Sick Children, Toronto, ON, Canada
e-mail: manokamna.agarwal@sickkids.ca

S. S. M. Fung
Department of Ophthalmology, University of California, Los Angeles, CA, USA
e-mail: SimonFung@mednet.ucla.edu

K. Mireskandari · A. Ali (✉)
Department of Ophthalmology and Vision Sciences, Hospital for Sick Children, Toronto, ON, Canada

Department of Ophthalmology and Vision Sciences, University of Toronto, Toronto, ON, Canada
e-mail: kamiar.mireskandari@sickkids.ca; asim.ali@utoronto.ca

A. Traish, V. P. Douglas (eds.), *Pediatric Ocular Surface Disease*,
https://doi.org/10.1007/978-3-031-30562-7_6

Table 6.1 Complications of HSCT. "Data taken from Bazinet et al. [5]"

Pre-engraftment complications (from start of conditioning regimen to neutrophil recovery)	Pancytopenia, gastrointestinal tract toxicities, infections, and organ dysfunction
Early post-engraftment complications (from neutrophil recovery to post-transplantation day 100)	Acute GVHD manifesting as skin rash, watery diarrhea, nausea or vomiting, jaundice, and abnormal liver function tests
Late post-engraftment complications (day 100 and beyond)	Chronic GVHD affecting the skin, and salivary and lacrimal glands, resulting in sicca syndrome. Pulmonary, gastrointestinal tract, and liver involvement. Increased risk of opportunistic infections in patients with chronic GVHD

HSCT hematopoietic stem cell transplantation, *GVHD* graft-versus-host disease.

suggested that there is a global increase of autologous HSCTs by 6.2% and allogeneic HSCTs by 7.0% over a 10-year period [3].

Prior to HSCT, the patient receives conditioning chemoradiotherapy to eliminate underlying hematologic malignant cells and sufficiently suppress host immunity to permit successful engraftment of donor HSCs. To enhance engraftment and reduce the risk of recurrent infections, donor T cells are infused along with the HSCs. However, the infused donor T cells recognize the host cells as foreign and attack the epithelial cells of various organs leading to graft-versus-host disease (GVHD) [4]. In allogenic HSCT, GVHD is an important cause of post-transplant morbidity and mortality in otherwise well-engrafted patients. Complications associated with HSCT are enumerated in Table 6.1.

Peripheral Blood Versus Bone Marrow HSCT

About 70% of adult and 30% of pediatric allogeneic HSCT are performed using hematopoietic progenitor cells obtained from the peripheral blood of an unrelated donor [6]. In the pediatric population, bone marrow still continues to be the preferred source of HSCs [7]. In general, peripheral blood-mobilized HSCs are preferred as they have faster engraftment and less infectious complications than in bone marrow grafts due to higher numbers of CD34+ HSCs [8]. They also have a 10-time higher concentration of T cells, monocytes, and natural killer cells compared to a bone marrow graft. But this higher concentration of T cells in the peripheral blood HSC grafts correlates with a higher incidence of GVHD in both related and unrelated HSCT [8, 9]. In contrast, the bone marrow graft has fewer T cells, correlating with a lower incidence of chronic GVHD in the unrelated-donor setting, although the graft failure rate is higher at 9%. In a systematic review and meta-analysis comparing allogeneic bone marrow transplantation and peripheral blood stem cell transplantation in children, five-year overall survival was similar between the two groups. However, the incidence of chronic GVHD was higher in the peripheral blood HSCT group (35.4%) compared to the bone marrow transplant group (20.2%). There was no significant between-group difference in incidences of acute GVHD (32.7% versus 24.9%) [10].

Graft-Versus-Host Disease (GVHD)

GVHD is a multisystem allogeneic immune response characterized by dysregulation of the immune system and impairment of organ function, leading to increased mortality rates in patients receiving HSCT [11]. Almost 40–60% of those undergoing allogeneic HSCT can develop GVHD [12]. GVHD shares similar clinical features to Sjogren syndrome, scleroderma, primary biliary cirrhosis, bronchiolitis obliterans, immune cytopenias, and chronic immunodeficiency [7]. The primary cells responsible for acute GVHD are donor T-helper type 1 cells that recognize the host antigens in skin, liver, and GI tract. In chronic GVHD, donor T-helper type 2 cells mediate infiltration of skin, lungs, liver, GI tract, oral mucosa, and/or eyes. The degree of HLA mismatch correlates with the severity of GVHD.

Classification of GVHD

According to the National Institutes of Health (NIH) Working Group, GVHD is classified as acute or chronic based on clinical manifestations rather than the time since onset of GVHD. Acute GVHD is divided into the classic form and late-onset acute GVHD. Classic acute GVHD occurs within 100 days of HSCT and manifests as maculopapular rash (skin involvement is seen in almost 80% cases), gastrointestinal tract symptoms (54% patients have GI tract involvement), or cholestatic hepatitis (51% have liver involvement). The persistent, recurrent, or late-onset acute GVHD occurs beyond 100 days of HSCT with features of acute GVHD. Chronic GVHD includes classic chronic GVHD and overlap syndrome. Classic chronic GVHD lacks features or characteristics of acute GVHD and affects multiple organs with skin the most commonly involved in almost 75% of patients. Oral mucosa and salivary glands, liver and eyes are also commonly involved in almost 30–60% patients. In overlap syndrome, diagnostic features of chronic GVHD and acute GVHD appear together [13].

Ocular GVHD

Incidence

Ocular GVHD can occur in 40–60% of patients after allogeneic HSCT and in some, it can be the initial presentation of systemic GVHD. Some studies have reported incidences as high as 90%. This discrepancy in incidence rate is due to the use of different diagnostic criteria for reporting ocular GVHD. Ocular involvement is more commonly seen in chronic GVHD (in greater than 50% of patients) compared to acute GVHD (approximately 10% of patients) [14].

In a recent study by Pellegrini et al., the incidence of ocular GVHD was 20% at 1 year, 30% at 2 years, 40% at 3 years, 47% at 4 years, and 50% at 5 years [15]. Review of the previous literature indicates a paucity in available data on pediatric ocular GVHD. Many authors have reported ocular complications in children undergoing bone marrow transplant, but until recently none has reported the incidence of ocular GVHD. In 2021, Hébert et al. reported that 39% children developed ocular GVHD after having systemic GVHD [16]. Jeppesen et al. recently published data on the incidence of ocular GVHD in pediatric HSCT, consisting of 484 consecutive children receiving HSCTs from 1980 to 2016. The cumulative incidence was 1.9% for acute ocular GVHD, 6.0% for chronic ocular GVHD, 8.7% for new onset DED, and 12.7% for new onset corneal fluorescein staining among children less than 18 years of age undergoing allogeneic HSCT [17]. Other studies are detailed in Table 6.2.

Risk Factors

Understanding the risk factors for systemic and ocular GVHD is important in preventing complications associated with the disease. Many studies identify higher recipient age as a significant risk factor for chronic as well as ocular GVHD [15, 29]. The use of peripheral blood as a source of HSCs and prior acute GVHD are also associated with an increased risk of chronic and ocular GVHD [15]. Recently, Hébert et al. studied the risk factors for ocular involvement in pediatric GVHD. They noted that children suffering from cutaneous or pulmonary GVHD showed an increased risk of ocular GVHD ($p = 0.03$ and 0.02, respectively). Also, children with multi-organ GVHD had a significantly increased risk of ocular GVHD ($p = 0.05$) [16]. Jeppesen et al. found that busulfan was a risk factor for developing acute ocular GVHD, and malignant disease for developing new corneal fluorescein staining [17]. Older studies have identified acute lymphoblastic leukemia (ALL), acute myeloid leukemia (AML), thrombocytopenia, and Wiskott-Aldrich syndrome as risk factors for ocular GVHD in children [25, 27]. The signs and symptoms of ocular GVHD are discussed in Table 6.3.

Table 6.2 Available studies on pediatric ocular GVHD/ocular complications after HSCT

Author/year	Type of study	Aim of the study	Total number and age of participants	Time from transplant to development of oGVHD or ocular complications	Ocular complications	Signs	Treatments received
Jeppesen et al. (2022) [17]	RO	To describe the incidence & risk factors for oGVHD and DED in children undergoing HSCT with a long follow-up period	484 consecutive children <16 years of age	Median time to acute oGVHD diagnosis was 38 days (range 8–122) Chronic oGVHD was 1056 days post-transplant (range 134–4122)	Acute oGVHD noted in 9/418 Chronic oGVHD noted in 26/418	Used criteria for acute oGVHD by Jabs et al. [18] and International Consensus Criteria for ocular cGVHD for chronic oGVHD [19]	–
Hébert et al. (2021) [16]	RO	To identify risk factors for oGVHD in children with GVHD	38 children aged <18 years	683 ± 866 days (range: 11–2594 days)	39% (15/38)	Blepharitis (3/15) Punctate epithelial erosions (6/15) Cataract (5/15) Conjunctival hyperemia (5/15) Reduced tear (10/15)	Artificial tears (9/15) Topical cyclosporin (2/15) Topical steroids (1/15) Punctal plugs (1/15)
Kızıltunç et al. (2021) [20]	RO	To evaluate frequency & findings of dry eye associated with ocular graft-versus-host disease (GVHD)	218 patients aged 3–18 years	–	Chronic oGVHD 30/ 47 patients (63.8%)	Dry eye syndrome	Preservative-free artificial tears (30/30) Topical cyclosporin A (4/30) Punctal plugs (1/30)

(continued)

Table 6.2 (continued)

Hoehn et al. (2020) [21]	RO	To determine the ocular complications in children & adolescents surviving at least 1 year post HSCT	162 patients aged 7–18 years	–	–	Cataract (57/162) Dry eye syndrome (51/162) oGVHD (2/162) Herpes zoster ophthalmicus (6/162) Infectious retinitis (6/162)	Cataract surgery (4/162)
Hoehn et al. (2018) [22]	RO	To investigate ocular complications of HSCT	91 children aged <7 years	–	–	Cataract 37/91 Punctate epithelial erosions(11/91) Reduced tear (2/91) Preseptal cellulitis (2/91) Herpes simplex keratitis (1/91) Conjunctivitis (1/91) Corneal haze (1/91) Optic nerve atrophy (6/91) Ocular chloromas (2/91) Retinoblastoma (1/91) Presumed ocular histoplasmosis syndrome (1/91) Atrophic retinal holes (1/91) Retinal hemorrhage (1/91) Chorioretinal scar (1/91)	Cataract surgery (8/91) Acyclovir (1/91) Penetrating Keratoplasty (1/91)
Ayuso et al. (2013) [23]	P	To study the development of ocular complications In children within 1 year after HSCT	49 consecutive patients aged <18	Ocular complications median time was first 3 months, and dry eye was 5 months	27% (13/49) developed ocular complications	DED 7/14 Subretinal hemorrhage 6/12 Optic disc edema 3/6 Chorioretinal lesions 2/4 Vitritis 1/ 2 Raised intra ocular pressure 1/ 2	

Kinori et al. (2015) [24]	P	To evaluate if HSCT without TBI had lower or milder ocular complication rates in pediatric population	33 children aged 0–18 years	cGVHD development 12 months (range 2–24 months)	Ocular involvement in 35% participants (8/23)	Dry eye 8/8 Recurrent erosions 1/8 Herpes zoster ophthalmicus 1/8 PSC cataract 1/8 Corneal abscess 1/8	Punctal plugs 3/8 Fortified topical antibiotics 1/8 Systemic valacyclovir and topical acyclovir and dexamethasone 1/8 Cataract surgery 1/8
Fahnehjelm et al. (2007) [25]	CS	To report prevalence of DED in children treated with HSCT	60 children aged 2–18 years	–	37/60	Staining <1–10% of the corneal surface in 29/37 Staining ≥10–25% of the corneal surface in 8/37	Lubricants 8/8 Topical corticosteroid 3/8 Topical cyclosporin A 2/8 Punctal plugs 3/8
Bradfield et al. (2005) [26]	RO	Rate and type of ocular complications, including those requiring ocular surgery, were analyzed	74 children aged 4 months to 18 years	1 year complication rate 16%	Ocular complications in 20.2% participants (15/74)	PSC 5/15 oGVHD 3/15 Corneal ulcer 1/15 CMV retinitis 2/15 Strabismus 2/15 Preseptal cellulitis 1/15 Conjunctivitis 1/15 Lymphoproliferative disorder 1/15 Transient visual loss 1/15	Lensectomy 2/15 Tarsorrhaphy for corneal ulcer 1/15 Iris biopsy 1/15
Suh et al. (1999) [27]	RO	To determine the prevalence & types of ocular abnormalities following BMT	104 consecutive patients aged <18 years		Ocular abnormalities in 51% patients (53/104)	PSC 24/53 DED 13/53 Posterior segment changes 14/53	

(continued)

Table 6.2 (continued)

| Ng et al. (1999) [28] | CS | To investigate ocular complications in BMT patients | 29 pediatric patients aged 1.5–15 years | 20.2 months (range 3–54 months) | – | Tear abnormality noted in 51.7% (15/29) Subconjunctival fibrosis 6.9% (2/15) Dry and scaly skin of the eyelids (1/15) Lens opacities (2/6 irradiated patients and 2/23 of non-irradiated patients) Fundus changes (2/15) | – |

oGVHD ocular graft-versus-host disease, *cGVHD* chronic graft-versus-host disease, *HSCT* hematopoietic stem cell transplantation, *DED* dry eye disease, *PSC* posterior subcapsular cataract, *BMT* bone marrow transplant, *TBI* total body irradiation, *RO* retrospective observational study, *P* prospective study, *CS* Cross-sectional study

Table 6.3 Signs and symptoms of ocular GVHD

Acute ocular GVHD	• Conjunctival involvement (almost 12–17% of patients) presenting as conjunctival hyperemia, chemosis, pseudomembranous conjunctivitis with/without ulcerative or hemorrhagic changes, and persistent corneal epithelial defects in severe cases
Chronic ocular GVHD	• Keratoconjunctivitis sicca (KCS) (almost 40–60% of patients) presenting as eye fatigue, dry eye or foreign body sensation, eye pain, photophobia, redness, burning, or itching in the eyes acute conjunctival inflammation and pseudomembranous and cicatricial conjunctivitis. Complications such as corneal epithelial defects, corneal ulcers, perforation, corneal neovascularization, limbal stem cell deficiency, and ultimately vision loss. Lid deformities in the form of cicatricial ectropion or entropion and trichiasis. Spontaneous lacrimal punctal occlusion

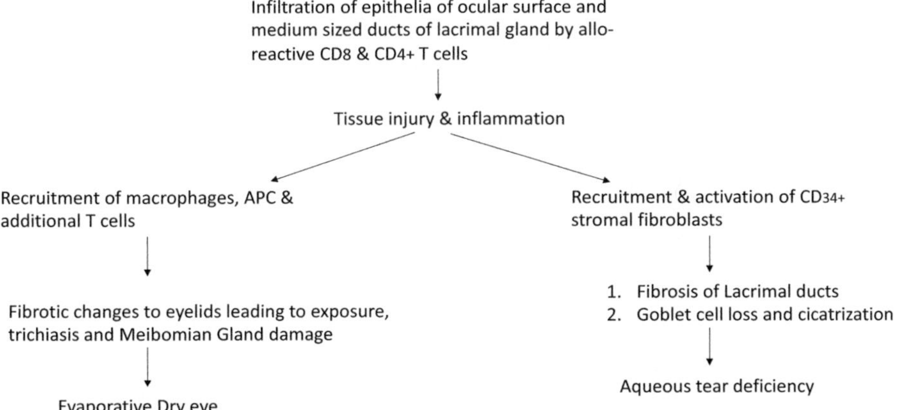

Fig. 6.1 Pathogenesis of dry eye in ocular GVHD. "Data taken from Carreno-Galeano et al [30]"

Histopathology

The immune response of ocular GVHD is T-cell mediated against the host tissue. There is infiltration of immune cells and inflammation of the ocular surface structures including the lacrimal gland, eyelids, cornea, and conjunctiva. Proliferating T cells cause localized ocular immune response manifesting as conjunctivitis. Infiltration of donor lymphocytes in the lacrimal gland leads to a widespread fibrosis and aqueous tear deficiency [30] (Fig. 6.1). Inflammation, reduced tear production, and increased evaporation lead to a high tear osmolarity and elevated cytokines (IL-6, IL-8, IL-17, IFN-g, TNF-a) and chemokines (CXCL8 and CXCL10) [31, 32].

On histopathology, total separation of the epithelium in the conjunctiva is noted in these patients. There is a decrease in goblet cells, necrosis of the epithelial cells, lymphocyte exocytosis and satellitosis, dyskeratotic cells, and formation of subepithelial microvesicles [18]. The lacrimal gland shows infiltration of T cells in the periductal areas, accumulation of a periodic acid-Schiff (PAS)-positive material in the acini and the ductules, and an increased number of stromal fibroblasts in the tissue [33]. In vivo confocal microscopy shows the infiltration of immune cells and dendritic cells in the subbasal nerves of the cornea [34]. Increased tear fluid extracellular DNA is also noted in ocular GVHD [35].

Diagnostic Criteria for Ocular GVHD

Acute Ocular GVHD

As conjunctivital involvement is predominantly seen in acute ocular GVHD, the disease severity is assessed by grading the conjunctivitis as follows [36]:

Stage 0: None
Stage 1: Hyperemia
Stage 2: Hyperemia with serosanguinous discharge
Stage 3: Pseudomembranous conjunctivitis
Stage 4: Pseudomembranous conjunctivitis with corneal epithelial sloughing

Chronic Ocular GVHD

In 2013, the International Chronic Ocular Graft-vs-Host-Disease (GVHD) Consensus Group proposed a diagnostic criteria for ocular GVHD. They identified 4 subjective and objective variables: Ocular Surface Disease Index (OSDI), Schirmer's test without anesthesia, corneal staining, and conjunctival injection. Each variable was scored 0–2 or 0–3, with a maximum composite score of 11. Consideration was also given to the presence or absence of systemic GVHD. On the basis of their composite score and the presence or absence of systemic GVHD, patients were assigned to one of three diagnostic categories (Table 6.4) [19, 37].

The National Institutes of Health (NIH) Consensus Development Project on Criteria for Clinical Trials in chronic GVHD established diagnostic criteria for ocular GVHD in 2005. It enumerated new onset dry, gritty or painful eyes, cicatricial conjunctivitis, keratoconjunctivitis sicca, and confluent areas of punctate keratopathy as distinctive signs, but insufficient alone to establish a diagnosis of chronic GVHD. Other features like photophobia, periorbital hyperpigmentation, difficulty in opening eyes in the morning due to mucoid secretions, and blepharitis are also noted. But the diagnosis of chronic GVHD is based on Schirmer's test results rather than the other clinical signs or symptoms of dry eye. Involvement of at least 1 organ with new onset ocular sicca, documented by a Schirmer's test value less than or equal to 5 mm at 5 min in both eyes, or a new onset keratoconjunctivitis sicca on slit lamp examination with a Schirmer's test value of 6–10 mm is sufficient for the diagnosis of chronic GVHD [13]. Conjunctival biopsy and histopathology can also aid in the diagnosis of ocular GVHD.

Table 6.4 The International Chronic Ocular Graft-vs-Host-Disease (GVHD) Consensus Group proposed diagnostic criteria for ocular GVHD. "Reproduced with permission from Ogawa et al [19]"

Severity scale in chronic ocular GVHD				
Severity score (points)	Schirmer's test (mm)	CFS (points)	OSDI (points)	Conj (points)
0	>15	0 (no staining)	<13	None
1	11–15	<2 (minimal staining)	13–22	Mild/ moderate
2	6–10	2–3 (mild/ moderate staining)	23–32	Severe
3	≤5	≥4 (severe staining)	≥33	

Severity classification; Total score (points); (Schirmer's test score + CFS score + OSDI score + Conj injection score) = none; 0–4, mild/moderate; 5–8, severe, 9–11

Diagnosis of chronic ocular GVHD			
Diagnosis	None (points)	Probable oGVHD (points)	Definite oGVHD (points)
Systemic GVHD (−)	0–5	6–7	≥8
Systemic GVHD (+)	0–3	4–5	≥6

CFS Corneal fluorescein staining, *OSDI* Ocular Surface Disease Index, *Conj* Conjunctival injection, *oGVHD* ocular GVHD.

In children, corneal fluorescein staining and the Schirmer's test should be given more weightage compared to the OSDI index for, as seen with other studies on dry eye diseases in children, questionnaires are less reliable in this age group [38, 39].

Non-GVHD Ocular Complications

Children undergoing HSCT can present with additional ocular complications even without ocular GVHD. This is attributed to the treatment received before and/or after HSCT. Lens opacification in the form of subcapsular cataracts is the most common ocular complication. Almost 70% of the children receiving total body irradiation and corticosteroids for allo-HSCT develop cataracts. Medications received by children after HSCT can also cause ocular toxicity. Cytosine arabinoside can commonly cause keratoconjunctivitis or ocular pain and foreign body sensation. Imatinib can lead to periorbital edema. Corticosteroids are well known to cause cataracts and raised intraocular pressure. Preventive therapy in the form of systemic antihistamines and anticholinergics can exacerbate the ocular GVHD by reducing lacrimal secretions. Systemic use of busulfan, carmustine, and cyclosporine can also lead to ischemic microvascular retinopathy in 0–10% of patients. Due to this high incidence rate and possible amblyogenic effects because of cataracts, children,

Table 6.5 Non-GVHD complications after HSCT. "Data taken from Inamoto et al [41]"

Cataract	Posterior subcapsular cataract due to total body irradiation and corticosteroids (noted in 11–100% adults and 4–76% children)
Bacterial infections	Gram positive or gram negative keratitis due to neutropenia and impaired immunity (in <2% patients)
Fungal infections	Candida or aspergillus keratitis or endophthalmitis due to immunosuppression (in <2% patients)
Viral infections	CMV retinitis (in <1–5% patients) can also lead to retinal detachment in 1% of patients, HSV and VZV (rare)
Glaucoma	Noted in 0.4–1.7% patients
Central retinal vein occlusion	Rare
Retinal hemorrhages	Noted in 3.2% patients due to thrombocytopenia

GVHD graft-versus-host disease, *CMV* cytomegalovirus, *HSV* herpes simplex virus, *VZV* varicella-zoster virus

especially under the age of 8 years should undergo periodic ophthalmic evaluation after HSCT for every 6–12 months [40]. As these children will require cataract surgery, intraoperative precautions should be taken to minimize surface damage. These include frequent irrigation with BSS or use of viscoelastic to avoid epithelial damage. Other non-GVHD ocular complications as reviewed by Inamoto et al. in 2018 have been listed below (Table 6.5).

Preventive Measures and Screening Strategies

There are currently no preventive therapies for ocular GVHD. It is imperative to perform periodic ophthalmic examinations in children who undergo HSCT at baseline and after HSCT by a pediatric ophthalmologist with experience in GVHD. The latest report by the Ancillary Therapy and Supportive Care Working Group recommends photoprotection and surveillance for infection, cataract formation, and increased intraocular pressure every 3–12 months and after immunosuppressive therapy is completed during extended survivorship [41].

Treatment Strategies

Acute Ocular GVHD

The goal of treatment for ocular GVHD is to reduce inflammation, optimize the ocular surface, and stabilize the tear film. Acute ocular GVHD should be managed with the aim to reduce ongoing ocular surface inflammation and thereby prevent long-term complications of KCS and cicatrization. Mild ocular GVHD is treated with topical therapy, whereas systemic immunosuppression is considered for patients with a moderate to severe NIH global score. In stage 3 and 4, acute ocular GVHD-related conjunctivitis, aggressive topical steroid, and removal of inflammatory membranes or pseudomembranes may improve the rate of epithelial healing and decrease scarring [42]. Frequent instillation of preservative-free lubricants dilutes the inflammatory cytokines and chemokines. In the case of corneal involvement, topical antibiotics can be started to prevent secondary complications.

Chronic Ocular GVHD

The goal of treatment for chronic ocular GVHD revolves around reduction of symptoms and signs caused by three changes: lacrimal gland dysfunction leading to aqueous tear deficiency, meibomian gland dysfunction altering the lipid layer, and corneo-conjunctival inflammation leading to the loss of goblet cells and mucous deficiency [43]. Having a step-wise approach helps in management of chronic ocular GVHD. Maintaining a balance between increasing immunosuppression and graft-versus-tumor effect is essential in keeping patients in a cancer-free remission state [44]. The paucity of literature on pediatric ocular GVHD management and lack of controlled trials makes management decisions difficult, and sometimes the treatment strategies recommended for adults are not well-suited for children. With the same level of dry eye disease, children have fewer symptoms compared to adults [45]. Use of dry eye questionnaires like the OSDI is difficult in younger children and these not validated for this age group. Treatment includes medical (local and systemic) and surgical therapies.

Addressing Aqueous Tear Deficiency

Lubricants have been the mainstay of ocular GVHD treatment. It is advisable to use preservative-free and phosphate-free lubricating eye drops to avoid corneal calcification and cytotoxicity [19]. Although lubricants have the theoretical benefit of diluting inflammatory mediators and providing symptomatic relief, they do not address ongoing ocular surface inflammation. In conjunction with ointments, environmental modifications like humidifiers in dry indoor spaces and moisture goggles at night can help keep the ocular surface hydrated. Permanent or temporary punctal occlusion in the form of punctal cautery or plugs can help preserve residual tears. Figure 6.2 Occluding the puncta also results in eye drop retention for a longer period in the eyes which can reduce the frequency of lubricant instillation [44, 46]. In children, limited cooperation at the slit lamp may compel the surgeon to perform the procedure under anesthesia. A study by Mataftsi et al. on the use of punctal plugs in children with dry eyes reported that almost 70% required general anesthesia [47]. Scleral lenses have also shown to be effective in providing symptomatic relief and protection to the ocular surface in ocular GVHD [48]. Custom-designed scleral

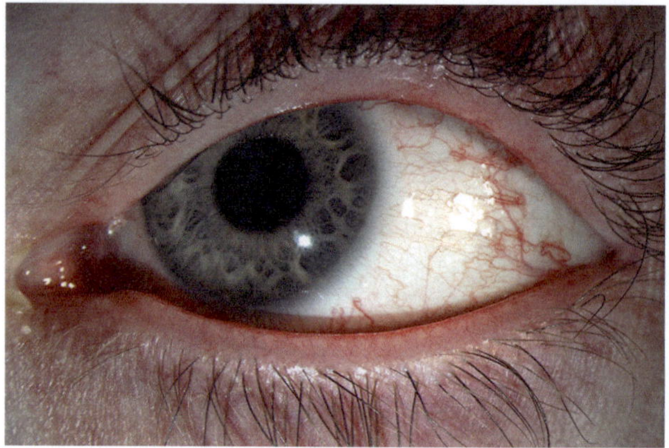

Fig. 6.2 A 16 year old with chronic ocular GVHD and moderate aqueous tear deficiency. Managed with punctal plugs and topical cyclosporine 0.05%

lenses have been successfully used in pediatric patients under 13 years of age with severe ocular surface diseases [49]. Younger patients may require assistance with lens insertion and removal. There may also be a high cost associated with these customized lenses [50].

Newer therapeutic options in the form of autologous blood component eye drops have also shown encouraging results in GVHD patients. These include 50% autologous serum tear drops, platelet-rich plasma (PRP) eye drops, as well as plasma rich in growth factors (PRGF) eye drops [51–53]. These are all rich in growth factors important for corneal and conjunctival integrity. However, the use of autologous blood might not be possible in younger patients. In such cases, allogeneic serum (from parents or siblings) can serve as an alternative and have been reported as effective in chronic GVHD [54, 55]. The use of 20% umbilical cord serum eye drops is also reported in GVHD. Compared to autologous serum, the advantages of using umbilical cord serum are that a large amount can be obtained at once from the umbilical vein and that the same sample may serve many patients [56].

Addressing Ocular Surface Inflammation

Topical corticosteroids not only reduce the inflammation by preventing cellular migration and phagocytosis, but also by preventing cicatrization. Prednisolone acetate 1% is often used 3–4 times per day. Side effects of topical corticosteroids are well known. They should be used with caution in patients with epithelial defects or ulceration. Preferring a lower potency steroid in mild ocular GVHD-related inflammation can reduce the risks of cataracts and secondary glaucoma in these children. As an alternative to corticosteroids, the use of selective calcineurin inhibitors like topical cyclosporin 0.05% and tacrolimus 0.03% for ocular GVHD is well established in moderate to severe ocular GVHD [57, 58]. Though the studies with cyclosporin and tacrolimus in GVHD included some pediatric patients, there is no exclusive data on pediatric ocular GVHD management with calcineurin inhibitors [57, 58].

Addressing Meibomian Gland Dysfunction (MGD)

Mild to moderate MGD may benefit from conventional therapy including lid hygiene, warm compresses, and lid massage. Topical antibiotics like bacitracin or erythromycin ointment can be applied on the lid margins at bedtime. If topical antibiotics are insufficient, oral erythromycin (one-quarter to a full-strength dose of 50 mg/kg/day) can be used in patients younger than 8 years of age, and doxycycline (50 mg b.i.d) in patients over 8 years of age [59]. Flaxseed oil can be used to supplement omega-3 essential fatty acids in children [60].

Surgical Management of Ocular GVHD

Surgical intervention is performed for complications of ocular GVHD or to enhance the protection of eye. Filamentary keratitis can be managed by epithelial debridement. Multilayer amniotic membrane transplantation may be considered an alternative for reconstructing the ocular surface in GVHD [61, 62]. Tarsorrhaphy has proven effective in the treatment of severe keratoconjunctivitis sicca by reducing surface exposure [63] (Fig. 6.3). Cases presenting with corneal melts or perforation require urgent tectonic keratoplasty to restore the globe integrity. Though uncommon, limbal stem cell deficiency (LSCD) may also be related to ocular GVHD [64]. In adults, successful conjunctival limbal allograft has been performed for LSCD due to GVHD by using same HLA-identical bone marrow transplantation donor [65]. No reports on management of GVHD-associated LSCD could be found in children. Rarely, chronic conjunctival inflammation can lead to progressive conjunctival scarring which later results in entropion or trichiasis, requiring surgical correction [66] (Fig. 6.4).

In summary, GVHD should be managed in a multi-disciplinary fashion. The role of an experienced ophthalmologist cannot be understated in the management of ocular GVHD. Children scheduled to undergo HSCT should have a baseline ophthalmic examination to rule out pre-existing ocular conditions including dry eyes, and thereafter have a comprehensive periodic ocular evaluation. Early diagnosis

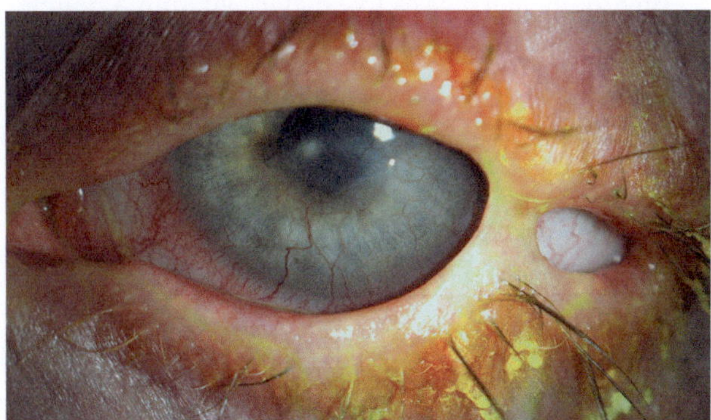

Fig. 6.3 A 14 year old with ocular and cutaneous GVHD, corneal neovascularization, severe aqueous tear deficiency, cataract, and a stretched tarsorrhaphy scar

Fig. 6.4 An 11 year old with end stage cicatrization due to ocular GVHD with keratinization of the ocular surface and ankyloblepharon

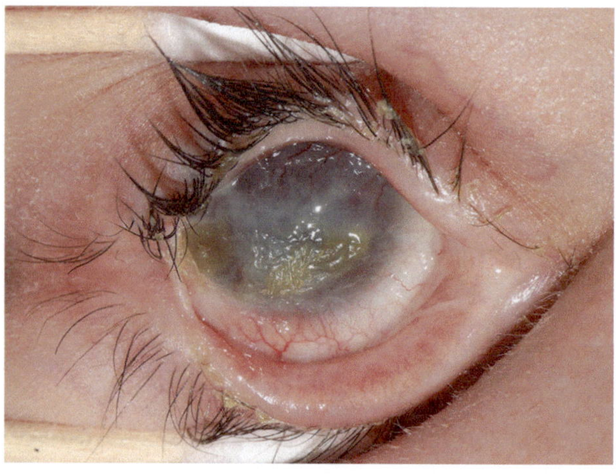

with prompt and aggressive treatment will help in preventing irreversible long-term complications of HSCT.

Other Causes of Dry Eye in Pediatric Patients

Dry eye is rare in children, and diagnosis is often overlooked. Apart from GVHD, it can be associated with various pediatric diseases like [67]:

1. Congenital disorders like (a) familial dysautonomia (Riley-Day syndrome) presenting as corneal anesthesia and alacrima; (b) allgrove syndrome (Triple-A syndrome) manifesting as adrenocorticotropic hormone (ACTH) resistant adrenal insufficiency, alacrima, and achalasia; (c) congenital alacrima; (d) congenital corneal anesthesia; (e) cystic fibrosis; and (f) ectodermal dysplasia.
2. Autoimmune and inflammatory diseases including (a) Sjogren syndrome; (b) graft-versus-host disease; (c) Stevens-Johnson syndrome; (d) vernal keratoconjunctivitis; and (e) juvenile rheumatoid arthritis.
3. Environmental causes like dietary vitamin A deficiency and chronic use of medications like oral retinoids.

Eyelid disorders like ectropion, entropion, burns, tumors, and congenital lid defects leading to increased exposure and evaporation of tears.

Assessment of Dry Eyes in Children

Pediatric clinical studies have shown that children are less specific in describing their existing ocular surface discomfort. Most of the dry eye tests used in diagnosis and follow-up of dry eye in adults can also be performed in children after some adjustments according to their age [38, 39]. Examples of dry eye diagnostic tests that can be performed in children include Schirmer's test, ferning test, tear film osmolarity, corneal and conjunctival staining, tear break-up time, use of non-invasive imaging devices to document change in meibomian gland structure. Schirmer's test is reliable in measuring tear production in children as well as in infants [68]. Schirmer's test without anesthesia and with less than 10 mm of wetting after 5 min is considered abnormal. Alternatively, the phenol red test can also be performed instead of Schirmer's test [67]. The ferning test also helps in grading the dry eye. This test is performed by collecting one drop of tear from the lower lacrimal meniscus and placing it on a microscope slide which is allowed to dry by evaporation for 10 min. Ferning patterns include (1) uniform large arborization, (2) small abundant ferning, (3) incomplete/partial ferning, and (4) no ferning. Type 3 and 4 are related to dry eye [67]. Tear osmolarity though widely used as an indicator for dry eyes in adults is rarely used in children due to variability in results [38, 39]. One of the most reliable and valuable tests in diagnosing severity of dry eye in children is corneal fluorescein staining [69]. Fluorescein is a vital dye used to stain the ocular surface and evaluate the degree of corneal epitheliopathy. Lissamine green and rose bengal stains can also be used [70]. A reduction in tear break-up time (TBUT) can indicate instabilities in the tear film. It is a standard measurement for diagnosing dry eye in adults and is also clinically useful in children. A meta-analysis combining results from multiple studies estimates the TBUT to be 14.6 s in healthy children [71].

Very few studies have been done to date to assess dry eye status in children. There is definitely a lacuna when it comes to assessment of dry eye in pediatric population, and therefore reliability of these diagnostic tests in children is yet to be established. Attempts have been made by comparing the signs and symptoms of dry eye in children with autoimmune disorders like SLE and healthy children by using common dry eye assessment tools. It was noted that there was no difference in symptoms between the two groups. Dry eye assessment tests such as tear osmolarity, tear break-up time, Schirmer's test, and lissamine green staining were not statistically different between the two groups. It was important to note that corneal staining served as a statistically significant tool in comparing the two groups as 58% children with SLE had corneal staining compared to only 20% in healthy children [39]. Another study that included children with blepharokeratoconjunctivitis (BKC) also emphasized use of corneal fluorescein staining to distinguish BKC patients from healthy children [38]. In contrast, a study done comparing dry eye diagnostic tests between diabetic and healthy children showed higher tear film osmolarity, lower Schirmer's score, and changes in conjunctival cytology in diabetic children [72]. Despite these findings, we believe that use of corneal fluorescein staining is definitely most helpful in diagnosing children with dry eye.

Often, systemic findings also play an important role in the diagnosis of dry eye in children. Though rare at a young age, children can present with features of Sjogren syndrome (e.g., dry mouth) and further clinical examination can reveal associated red eye, photosensitivity, oral ulceration, periodontitis, or parotidomegaly. Such children should undergo a complete rheumatological/immunological assessment including C-reactive protein, anti-SSA, and anti-SSB [73].

It is also worthwhile to assess the meibomian glands in children, as even in the normal asymptomatic pediatric population, there can be meibomian gland alterations [74]. As in an older population, ethnic differences in morphology of meibomian gland were noted in Asian children compared to those with a Caucasian ethnicity. Asian children had a higher incomplete blink rate and inferior lid wiper epitheliopathy compared to Caucasian children. Yet there was no difference in tear film quality or dry eye symptoms. This study shows that meibomian gland disease is more prone to develop in particular ethnic groups compared to others [75]. Increased screen time is also associated with severe meibomian gland atrophy in children [76]. A Korean study reported a dry eye disease rate of 6.6% in children. There were 96.7% of children in the dry eye group who used smartphones compared to 55.4% in the control group. A significantly higher use of computers and lower outdoor activity time was noted in the dry eye group compared to controls. This study also presented a comparative analysis before and after cessation of smartphone use over 4 weeks for the dry eye group and found statistical improvement in tear break-up time, OSDI score, and corneal staining [77]. Increased screen time is also shown to be related to childhood obesity and learning disabilities in addition to dry eyes [78]. Increased screen time was also noted during the COVID-19 lockdown. A study has shown increase in SPEED questionnaire score in pediatric population after March 2020 compared to pre-Covid scores [79].

Conclusion

In summary, dry eye disease is not uncommon in children. It can be associated with congenital, environmental, or systemic conditions including graft-versus-host disease. Ophthalmologists should be aware that the signs of dry eye in children may present without any symptoms. Gaps in the literature in this area include a need for longitudinal, prospective studies on outcomes of dry in children and the need for pediatric normative data for dry eye diagnostic tests which will help determine which diagnostic criteria are best suited for children. Early diagnosis and treatment of dry eye disease in children can help in avoiding complications, improve comfort and quality of life.

References

1. Henig I, Zuckerman T. Hematopoietic stem cell transplantation—50 years of evolution and future perspectives. Rambam Maimonides Med J. 2014;5:e0028. https://doi.org/10.5041/rmmj.10162.
2. Snowden JA, Sharrack B, Akil M, Kiely DG, Lobo A, Kazmi M, et al. Autologous haematopoietic stem cell transplantation (aHSCT) for severe resistant autoimmune and inflammatory diseases–a guide for the generalist. Clin Med (Lond). 2018;18:329–34. https://doi.org/10.7861/clinmedicine.18-4-329.

3. Niederwieser D, Baldomero H, Bazuaye N, Bupp C, Chaudhri N, Corbacioglu S, et al. One and a half million hematopoietic stem cell transplants: continuous and differential improvement in worldwide access with the use of non-identical family donors. Haematologica. 2022;107:1045–53. https://doi.org/10.3324/haematol.2021.279189.

4. Dutt S, Tseng D, Ermann J, George TI, Liu YP, Davis CR, et al. Naive and memory T cells induce different types of graft-versus-host disease. J Immunol. 2007;179:6547–54. https://doi.org/10.4049/jimmunol.179.10.6547.

5. Bazinet A, Popradi G. A general practitioner's guide to hematopoietic stem-cell transplantation. Curr Oncol. 2019;26:187–91. https://doi.org/10.3747/co.26.5033.

6. Passweg JR, Baldomero H, Bader P, Bonini C, Cesaro S, Dreger P, et al. Hematopoietic SCT in Europe 2013: recent trends in the use of alternative donors showing more haploidentical donors but fewer cord blood transplants. Bone Marrow Transplant. 2015;50:476–82. https://doi.org/10.1038/bmt.2014.312.

7. Salhotra A, Nakamura R. Overview of hematopoietic cell transplantation. In: Cotliar JA, editor. Atlas of graft-versus-host disease approaches to diagnosis and treatment. Cham: Springer; 2017. p. 1–12.

8. Blaise D, Kuentz M, Fortanier C, Bourhis JH, Milpied N, Sutton L, et al. Randomized trial of bone marrow versus lenograstim-primed blood cell allogeneic transplantation in patients with early-stage leukemia: a report from the Société Française de Greffe de Moelle. J Clin Oncol. 2008;18:537–46. https://doi.org/10.1200/JCO.2000.18.3.537.

9. Anasetti C, Logan BR, Lee SJ, Waller EK, Weisdorf DJ, Wingard JR, et al. Peripheral-blood stem cells versus bone marrow from unrelated donors. N Engl J Med. 2012;367:1487–96. https://doi.org/10.1056/NEJMoa1203517.

10. Shimosato Y, Tanoshima R, Tsujimoto SI, Takeuchi M, Shiba N, Kobayashi T, et al. Allogeneic bone marrow transplantation versus peripheral blood stem cell transplantation for hematologic malignancies in children: a systematic review and meta-analysis. Biol Blood Marrow Transplant. 2020;26:88–93. https://doi.org/10.1016/j.bbmt.2019.07.025.

11. Ghimire S, Weber D, Mavin E, Wang XN, Dickinson AM, Holler E. Pathophysiology of GvHD and other HSCT-related major complications. Front Immunol. 2017;8:79. https://doi.org/10.3389/fimmu.2017.00079.

12. Jagasia M, Arora M, Flowers ME, Chao NJ, McCarthy PL, Cutler CS, et al. Risk factors for acute GVHD and survival after hematopoietic cell transplantation. Blood. 2012;119:296–307. https://doi.org/10.1182/blood-2011-06-364265.

13. Filipovich AH, Weisdorf D, Pavletic S, Socie G, Wingard JR, Lee SJ, et al. National Institutes of Health consensus development project on criteria for clinical trials in chronic graft-versus-host disease: I. Diagnosis and staging working group report. Biol blood marrow Transplant. 2005;11:945–56. https://doi.org/10.1016/j.bbmt.2005.09.004.

14. Kezic JM, Wiffen S, Degli-Esposti M. Keeping an 'eye' on ocular GVHD. Clin Exp Optom. 2022;105:135–42. https://doi.org/10.1080/08164622.2021.1971047.

15. Pellegrini M, Bernabei F, Barbato F, Arpinati M, Giannaccare G, Versura P, et al. Incidence, risk factors and complications of ocular graft-versus-host disease following hematopoietic stem cell transplantation. Am J Ophthalmol. 2021;227:25–34. https://doi.org/10.1016/j.ajo.2021.02.022.

16. Hébert M, Archambault C, Doyon C, Ospina LH, Robert MC. Risk factors for ocular involvement in pediatric graft-versus-host disease. Cornea. 2021;40:1158–64. https://doi.org/10.1097/ICO.0000000000002659.

17. Jeppesen H, Kielsen K, Siersma V, Lindegaard J, Julian HO, Heegaard S, et al. Ocular graft-versus-host disease and dry eye disease after pediatric haematopoietic stem cell transplantation-incidence and risk factors. Bone Marrow Transplant. 2022;57:487–98. https://doi.org/10.1038/s41409-022-01564-2.

18. Jabs DA, Wingard J, Green WR, Farmer ER, Vogelsang G, Saral R. The eye in bone marrow transplantation: III. Conjunctival graft-vs-host disease. Arch Ophthalmol. 1989;107:1343–8. https://doi.org/10.1001/archopht.1989.01070020413046.

19. Ogawa Y, Kim SK, Dana R, Clayton J, Jain S, Rosenblatt MI, et al. International chronic ocular graft-vs-host-disease (GVHD) consensus group: proposed diagnostic criteria for chronic GVHD (part I). Sci Rep. 2013;3:1–6. https://doi.org/10.1038/srep03419.
20. Kızıltunç PB, Büyüktepe TÇ, Yalçındağ FN, Ertem M, İnce E, İleri T, et al. Ocular findings of pediatric dry eye related to graft-versus-host disease. Turkish J Ophthalmol. 2021;51:134–8. https://doi.org/10.4274/tjo.galenos.2020.88137.
21. Hoehn ME, Vestal R, Calderwood J, Gannon E, Cook B, Rochester R, et al. Ocular complications in school-age children and adolescents after allogeneic bone marrow transplantation. Am J Ophthalmol. 2020;213:153–60. https://doi.org/10.1016/j.ajo.2020.01.025.
22. Hoehn ME, Calderwood J, Gannon E, Cook B, Rochester R, Hartford C, et al. Ocular complications in a young pediatric population following bone marrow transplantation. J AAPOS. 2018;22:102–6. https://doi.org/10.1016/j.jaapos.2017.10.010.
23. Ayuso VK, Hettinga Y, van der Does P, Boelens JJ, Rothova A, de Boer J. Ocular complications in children within 1 year after hematopoietic stem cell transplantation. JAMA Ophthalmol. 2013;131:470–5. https://doi.org/10.1001/jamaophthalmol.2013.2500.
24. Kinori M, Bielorai B, Souroujon D, Hutt D, Ben-Bassat Mizrachi I, Huna-Baron R. Ocular complications in children after hematopoietic stem cell transplantation without total body irradiation. Graefes Arch Clin Exp Ophthalmol. 2015;253:1397–402. https://doi.org/10.1007/s00417-015-2964-8.
25. Fahnehjelm KT, Törnquist AL, Winiarski J. Dry-eye syndrome after allogeneic stem-cell transplantation in children. Acta Ophthalmol. 2008;86:253–8. https://doi.org/10.1111/j.1600-0420.2007.01120.x.
26. Bradfield YS, Kushner BJ, Gangnon RE. Ocular complications after organ and bone marrow transplantation in children. J AAPOS. 2005;9:426–32. https://doi.org/10.1016/j.jaapos.2005.06.002.
27. Suh DW, Ruttum MS, Stuckenschneider BJ, Mieler WF, Kivlin JD. Ocular findings after bone marrow transplantation in a pediatric population. Ophthalmology. 1999;106:1564–70. https://doi.org/10.1016/S0161-6420(99)90454-2.
28. Ng JS, Lam DS, Li CK, Chik KW, Cheng GP, Yuen PM, et al. Ocular complications of pediatric bone marrow transplantation. Ophthalmology. 1999;106:160–4. https://doi.org/10.1016/S0161-6420(99)90023-4.
29. Ozawa S, Nakaseko C, Nishimura M, Maruta A, Cho R, Ohwada C, et al. Chronic graft-versus-host disease after allogeneic bone marrow transplantation from an unrelated donor: incidence, risk factors and association with relapse. A report from the Japan marrow donor program. Br J Haematol. 2007;137:142–51. https://doi.org/10.1111/j.1365-2141.2007.06543.x.
30. Carreno-Galeano JT, Dohlman TH, Kim S, Yin J, Dana R. A review of ocular graft-versus-host disease: pathophysiology, clinical presentation and management. Ocul Immunol Inflamm. 2021;29:1190–9. https://doi.org/10.1080/09273948.2021.1939390.
31. Na KS, Yoo YS, Hwang KY, Mok JW, Joo CK. Tear osmolarity and ocular surface parameters as diagnostic markers of ocular graft-versus-host disease. Am J Ophthalmol. 2015;160:143–9. https://doi.org/10.1016/j.ajo.2015.04.002.
32. Jung JW, Han SJ, Song MK, Kim EK, Min YH, Cheong JW, et al. Tear cytokines as biomarkers for chronic graft-versus-host disease. Biol Blood Marrow Transplant. 2015;21:2079–85. https://doi.org/10.1016/j.bbmt.2015.08.020.
33. Balaram M, Rashid S, Dana R. Chronic ocular surface disease after allogeneic bone marrow transplantation. Ocul Surf. 2005;3:203–10. https://doi.org/10.1016/s1542-0124(12)70207-0.
34. He J, Ogawa Y, Mukai S, Saijo-Ban Y, Kamoi M, Uchino M, et al. In vivo confocal microscopy evaluation of ocular surface with graft-versus-host disease-related dry eye disease. Sci Rep. 2017;7:10710–20. https://doi.org/10.1038/s41598-017-10237-w.
35. Tibrewal S, Sarkar J, Jassim SH, Gandhi S, Sonawane S, Chaudhary S, et al. Tear fluid extracellular DNA: diagnostic and therapeutic implications in dry eye disease. Invest Ophthalmol Vis Sci. 2013;54:8051–61. https://doi.org/10.1167/iovs.13-12844.
36. Shikari H, Antin JH, Dana R. Ocular graft-versus-host disease: a review. Surv Ophthalmol. 2013;58:233–51. https://doi.org/10.1016/j.survophthal.2012.08.004.

37. Tatematsu Y, Ogawa Y, Abe T, Kamoi M, Uchino M, Saijo-Ban Y, et al. Grading criteria for chronic ocular graft-versus-host disease: comparing the NIH eye score, Japanese dry eye score and DEWS 2007 score. Sci Rep. 2014;4:1–6. https://doi.org/10.1038/srep06680.

38. Elbaz U, Tone SO, Fung SS, Mireskandari K, Ali A. Evaluation of dry eye disease in children with blepharokeratoconjunctivitis. Can J Ophthalmol. 2022;57:98–104. https://doi.org/10.1016/j.jcjo.2021.02.017.

39. Tone SO, Elbaz U, Silverman E, Levy D, Williams S, Mireskandari K, et al. Evaluation of dry eye disease in children with systemic lupus erythematosus and healthy controls. Cornea. 2019;38:581–6. https://doi.org/10.1097/ICO.0000000000001902.

40. Inamoto Y, Valdés-Sanz N, Ogawa Y, Alves M, Berchicci L, Galvin J, et al. Ocular graft-versus-host disease after hematopoietic cell transplantation: expert review from the late effects and quality of life working committee of the CIBMTR and transplant complications working party of the EBMT. Biol Bone Marrow Transplant. 2019;54:662–73. https://doi.org/10.1038/s41409-018-0340-0.

41. Carpenter PA, Kitko CL, Elad S, Flowers ME, Gea-Banacloche JC, Halter JP, et al. National institutes of health consensus development project on criteria for clinical trials in chronic graft-versus-host disease: V. The 2014 Ancillary therapy and supportive care working group report. Biol Blood Bone Marrow Transplant. 2015;21:1167–87. https://doi.org/10.1016/j.bbmt.2015.03.024.

42. Kim SK, Couriel D, Ghosh S, Champlin R. Ocular graft vs. host disease experience from MD Anderson Cancer Center: newly described clinical spectrum and new approach to the management of stage III and IV ocular GVHD. Biol blood. Bone Marrow Transplant. 2006;12: 49–50.

43. Inamoto Y, Petriček I, Burns L, Chhabra S, DeFilipp Z, Hematti P, et al. Non-graft-versus-host disease ocular complications after hematopoietic cell transplantation: expert review from the late effects and quality of life working Committee of the Center for international blood and marrow transplant research and the transplant complications working Party of the European Society for blood and marrow transplantation. Biol Bone Marrow Transplant. 2019;25:e145–54. https://doi.org/10.1016/j.bbmt.2018.11.033.

44. Perez VL, Palioura S, Kim SK. Ocular graft-versus-host disease. In: Holland EJ, Mannis MJ, editors. Cornea: fundamentals, diagnosis and management. Ed 4 ed. Edinburgh: Elsevier; 2017.

45. Han SB, Yang HK, Hyon JY, Hwang JM. Children with dry eye type conditions may report less severe symptoms than adult patients. Graefes Arch Clin Exp Ophthalmol. 2012;251:791–6. https://doi.org/10.1007/s00417-012-2097-2.

46. Yaguchi S, Ogawa Y, Kamoi M, Uchino M, Tatematsu Y, Ban Y, et al. Surgical management of lacrimal punctal cauterization in chronic GVHD-related dry eye with recurrent punctal plug extrusion. Bone Marrow Transplant. 2012;47:1465–9. https://doi.org/10.1038/bmt.2012.50.

47. Mataftsi A, Subbu RG, Jones S, Nischal KK. The use of punctal plugs in children. Br J Ophthalmol. 2012;96:90–2. https://doi.org/10.1136/bjophthalmol-2011-300510.

48. Takahide K, Parker PM, Wu M, Hwang WY, Carpenter PA, Moravec C, Stehr B, et al. Use of fluid-ventilated, gas-permeable scleral lens for management of severe keratoconjunctivitis sicca secondary to chronic graft-versus-host disease. Biol Blood Marrow Transplant. 2007;13:1016–21. https://doi.org/10.1016/j.bbmt.2007.05.006.

49. Gungor İ, Schor K, Rosenthal P, Jacobs DS. The Boston scleral lens in the treatment of pediatric patients. J AAPOS. 2008;12:263–7. https://doi.org/10.1016/j.jaapos.2007.11.008.

50. Rathi VM, Mandathara PS, Vaddavalli PK, Srikanth D, Sangwan VS. Fluid filled scleral contact lens in pediatric patients: challenges and outcome. Contact Lens Ant Eye. 2012;35:189–92. https://doi.org/10.1016/j.clae.2012.03.001.

51. Ogawa Y, Okamoto S, Mori T, Yamada M, Mashima Y, Watanabe R, et al. Autologous serum eye drops for the treatment of severe dry eye in patients with chronic graft-versus-host disease. Bone Marrow Transplant. 2003;31:579–83. https://doi.org/10.1038/sj.bmt.1703862.

52. Sanchez-Avila RM, Merayo-Lloves J, Muruzabal F, Orive G, Anitua E. Plasma rich in growth factors for the treatment of dry eye from patients with graft versus host diseases. Eur J Ophthalmol. 2020;30:94–103. https://doi.org/10.1177/1120672118818943.

53. Alio JL, Rodriguez AE, Ferreira-Oliveira R, Wróbel-Dudzińska D, Abdelghany AA. Treatment of dry eye disease with autologous platelet-rich plasma: a prospective, interventional, non-randomized study. Ophthalmol Therapy. 2017;6:285–93. https://doi.org/10.1007/s40123-017-0100-z.
54. Na K-S, Kim MS. Allogeneic serum eye drops for the treatment of dry eye patients with chronic graft-versus-host disease. J Ocul Pharmacol Ther. 2012;28:479–83. https://doi.org/10.1089/jop.2012.0002.
55. Chiang C-C, Lin J-M, Chen W-L, Tsai Y-Y. Allogeneic serum eye drops for the treatment of severe dry eye in patients with chronic graft-versus-host disease. Cornea. 2007;26:861–3. https://doi.org/10.1097/ICO.0b013e3180645cd7.
56. Yoon KC, Jeong IY, Im SK, Park YG, Kim HJ, Choi J. Therapeutic effect of umbilical cord serum eyedrops for the treatment of dry eye associated with graft-versus-host disease. Bone Marrow Transplant. 2007;39:231–5. https://doi.org/10.1038/sj.bmt.1705566.
57. Ryu EH, Kim JM, Laddha PM, Chung E-S, Chung T-Y. Therapeutic effect of 0.03% tacrolimus ointment for ocular graft versus host disease and vernal keratoconjunctivitis. Korean J Ophthalmol. 2012;26:241–7. https://doi.org/10.3341/kjo.2012.26.4.241.
58. Lelli GJ, Musch DC, Gupta A, Farjo QA, Nairus TM, Mian SI. Ophthalmic cyclosporine use in ocular GVHD. Cornea. 2006;25:635–8. https://doi.org/10.1097/01.ico.0000208818.47861.1d.
59. Hammersmith KM. Blepharokeratoconjunctivitis in children. Curr Opin Ophthalmol. 2015;26:301–5. https://doi.org/10.1097/ICU.0000000000000167.
60. Jones SM, Weinstein JM, Cumberland P, Klein N, Nischal KK. Visual outcome and corneal changes in children with chronic blepharokeratoconjunctivitis. Ophthalmology. 2007;114:2271–80. https://doi.org/10.1016/j.ophtha.2007.01.021.
61. Peris-Martínez C, Menezo JL, Díaz-Llopis M, Aviñó-Martínez JA, Navea-Tejerina A, Risueño-Reguillo P. Multilayer amniotic membrane transplantation in severe ocular graft versus host disease. Eur J Ophthalmol. 2001;11:183–6. https://doi.org/10.1177/112067210101100215.
62. Peric Z, Skegro I, Durakovic N, Desnica L, Pulanic D, Serventi-Seiwerth R, et al. Amniotic membrane transplantation—a new approach to crossing the HLA barriers in the treatment of refractory ocular graft-versus-host disease. Bone Marrow Transplant. 2018;53:1466–9. https://doi.org/10.1038/s41409-018-0140-6.
63. Anderson NG, Regillo C. Ocular manifestations of graft versus host disease. Curr Opin Ophthalmol. 2004;15:503–7. https://doi.org/10.1097/01.icu.0000143684.22362.46.
64. Iyer G, Srinivasan B, Agarwal S, Agarwal M, Matai H. Surgical management of limbal stem cell deficiency. Asia Pac J Ophthalmol. 2020;9:512–23. https://doi.org/10.1097/APO.0000000000000326.
65. Cheung AY, Genereux BM, Auteri NJ, Sarnicola E, Govil A, Holland EJ. Conjunctival-limbal allografts in graft-versus-host disease using same HLA-identical bone marrow transplantation donor. Can J Ophthalmol. 2018;53:e120–2. https://doi.org/10.1016/j.jcjo.2017.09.004.
66. Dulz S, Wagenfeld L, Richard G, Schrum J, Muschol N, Keserü M. A case of a bilateral Cicatricial upper eyelid entropion after hematopoietic stem cell transplantation in Mucopolysaccharidosis type I. Ophthal Plast Reconstr Surg. 2017;33:S75–7. https://doi.org/10.1097/IOP.0000000000000592.
67. Alves M, Dias AC, Rocha EM. Dry eye in childhood: epidemiological and clinical aspects. Ocul Surf. 2008;6:44–51. https://doi.org/10.1016/s1542-0124(12)70104-0.
68. Dogru M, Karakaya H, Baykara M, Özmen A, Koksal N, Goto E, et al. Tear function and ocular surface findings in premature and term babies. Ophthalmology. 2004;111:901–5. https://doi.org/10.1016/j.ophtha.2003.07.017.
69. Baudouin C, Aragona P, Van Setten G, Rolando M, Irkeç M, del Castillo JB, et al. Diagnosing the severity of dry eye: a clear and practical algorithm. Br J Ophthalmol. 2014;98:1168–76. https://doi.org/10.1136/bjophthalmol-2013-304619.
70. Machado LM, Castro RS, Fontes BM. Staining patterns in dry eye syndrome: rose bengal versus lissamine green. Cornea. 2009;28:732–4. https://doi.org/10.1097/ICO.0b013e3181930c03.
71. Chidi-Egboka NC, Briggs NE, Jalbert I, Golebiowski B. The ocular surface in children: a review of current knowledge and meta-analysis of tear film stability and tear secretion in children. Ocul Surf. 2019;17:28–39. https://doi.org/10.1016/j.jtos.2018.09.006.

72. Gunay M, Celik G, Yildiz E, Bardak H, Koc N, Kirmizibekmez H, et al. Ocular surface characteristics in diabetic children. Curr Eye Res. 2016;41:1526–31. https://doi.org/10.310 9/02713683.2015.1136421.
73. Condé K, Guelngar CO, Barry MC, Atakla HG, Mohamed A, Cissé FA. Sjögren's syndrome in children: about 15 cases in Guinea Conakry. Eur J Med Res. 2021;26:66. https://doi.org/10.1186/s40001-021-00534-6.
74. Gupta PK, Stevens MN, Kashyap N, Priestley Y. Prevalence of Meibomian gland atrophy in a pediatric population. Cornea. 2018;37:426–30. https://doi.org/10.1097/ICO.0000000000001476.
75. Kim JS, Wang MTM, Craig JP. Exploring the Asian ethnic predisposition to dry eye disease in a pediatric population. Ocul Surf. 2019;17:70–7. https://doi.org/10.1016/j.jtos.2018.09.003.
76. Cremers SL, Khan AR, Ahn J, Cremers L, Weber J, Kossler AL, et al. New indicator of children's excessive electronic screen use and factors in meibomian gland atrophy. Am J Ophthalmol. 2021;229:63–70. https://doi.org/10.1016/j.ajo.2021.03.035.
77. Moon JH, Kim KW, Moon NJ. Smartphone use is a risk factor for pediatric dry eye disease according to region and age: a case control study. BMC Ophthalmol. 2016;16:188. https://doi.org/10.1186/s12886-016-0364-4.
78. Mineshita Y, Kim HK, Chijiki H, Nanba T, Shinto T, Furuhashi S, et al. Screen time duration and timing: effects on obesity, physical activity, dry eyes, and learning ability in elementary school children. BMC Public Health. 2021;21:422. https://doi.org/10.1186/s12889-021-10484-7.
79. Elhusseiny AM, Eleiwa TK, Yacoub MS, George J, ElSheikh RH, Haseeb A, et al. Relationship between screen time and dry eye symptoms in pediatric population during the COVID-19 pandemic. Ocul Surf. 2021;22:117–9. https://doi.org/10.1016/jtos.2021.08.002.

Chapter 7
Ophthalmic Manifestations of Stevens-Johnson Syndrome and Mycoplasma Induced Rash and Mucositis in Children

Abdelrahman M. Elhusseiny, Reem H. ElSheikh, and Hajirah N. Saeed

Introduction

Stevens-Johnson syndrome (SJS) and its more severe form, toxic epidermal necrolysis (TEN), are rare, life-threatening immune-mediated disorders affecting the skin and mucous membranes [1, 2]. Both SJS and TEN are considered variants within the same disease spectrum. The primary difference between them is the degree of total body surface area (TBSA) affected. Epidermal detachment that is <10% of TBSA is SJS, while >30% involvement of TBSA is TEN. Intermediate cases where epidermal detachment involves 10–30% of TBSA are considered SJS/TEN overlap syndrome [3]. Etiologic agents are often drugs such as antibiotics, non-steroidal

A. M. Elhusseiny
Department of Ophthalmology, Harvey and Bernice Jones Eye Institute, University of Arkansas for Medical Sciences, Little Rock, AR, USA

Department of Ophthalmology, Boston Children's Hospital, Harvard Medical School, Boston, MA, USA
e-mail: Abdelrahman.Elhusseiny@childrens.harvard.edu

R. H. ElSheikh
Department of Ophthalmology, Harvey and Bernice Jones Eye Institute, University of Arkansas for Medical Sciences, Little Rock, AR, USA

Department of Ophthalmology, Kasr Al-Ainy Hospitals, Cairo University, Cairo, Egypt

H. N. Saeed (✉)
Department of Ophthalmology, Illinois Eye and Ear Infirmary, University of Illinois at Chicago, Chicago, IL, USA

Department of Ophthalmology, Loyola University Medical Center, Maywood, IL, USA

Department of Ophthalmology, Massachusetts Eye and Ear, Harvard Medical School, Boston, MA, USA
e-mail: hnsaeed@uic.edu

© The Author(s), under exclusive license to Springer Nature Switzerland AG 2023
A. Traish, V. P. Douglas (eds.), *Pediatric Ocular Surface Disease*,
https://doi.org/10.1007/978-3-031-30562-7_7

anti-inflammatory drugs, and anticonvulsants, or, less commonly, infections. Mucocutaneous involvement in the setting of *Mycoplasma pneumoniae* (MP) infection was previously considered to be on the same spectrum as SJS/TEN or erythema multiforme [4–6]. In 2015, Canavan and colleagues described Mycoplasma pneumonia-induced rash and mucositis (MIRM) as a separate entity distinct from SJS/TEN. In MIRM, patients often have severe mucositis affecting multiple sites with less impressive skin involvement than SJS/TEN [7]. Several methods have been developed to improve the detection of MP, including the measurement of MP-specific antibody-secreting cells [8]. Other infectious agents have been noted to cause a disease process similar to MIRM, with the degree of mucosal involvement out of proportion to skin involvement. Accordingly, a recent classification has been proposed to define other infectious-related conditions as reactive infectious mucocutaneous eruptions (RIME) [9].

In this book chapter, we will discuss ocular involvement in pediatric SJS/TEN, MIRM, and RIME. There are relatively little data and, as such, no consensus on disease presentation and management in these rare disease entities in the pediatric population. This chapter will focus on the published literature and the authors' expert, practice-based opinion.

Stevens-Johnson Syndrome and Toxic Epidermal Necrolysis

SJS/TEN is more common in children than adults, affecting 36 individuals/million/year, as compared to 4–12 adult individuals/million/year [10]. While mortality rates are higher in adults compared to children (5–30% vs. 0–17%), the severity of ocular disease appears to be worse in children [11–14]. In the pediatric population, drug-induced SJS/TEN represents 72–90% of cases, with antibiotics and anticonvulsants the most commonly implicated drugs [15–18]. Up to 17% of cases are idiopathic [16, 19].

Ocular surface involvement is common in SJS/TEN, which, if not recognized early and left untreated, can result in significant ocular morbidity, including dry eye, limbal stem cell deficiency (LSCD), keratopathy, corneal scarring, and ocular surface keratinization [20–24]. In the acute phase of the disease, the incidence of ocular involvement may be up to 100% of cases in both children and adults [25, 26]. Chronic ocular sequelae can affect up to 75% of these patients [12, 27–29].

Few studies in the literature have exclusively studied ocular involvement in SJS/TEN in the pediatric population [28–30]. In a retrospective study conducted by Catt and colleagues [28] including 36 patients (20 had SJS, 7 had TEN, and 9 had overlap syndrome), 29/36 patients (81%) had acute ocular involvement with conjunctivitis being the most common presentation (78%) (Fig. 7.1). This was the earliest sign of acute ocular involvement together with subconjunctival hemorrhage (33%), and conjunctival membranes (28%), occurring within the first day of hospital admission. At a median of 3 days of hospital admission, 50% of patients had superficial punctate keratopathy, and 25% had epithelial defects. By the fourth week, 28% of

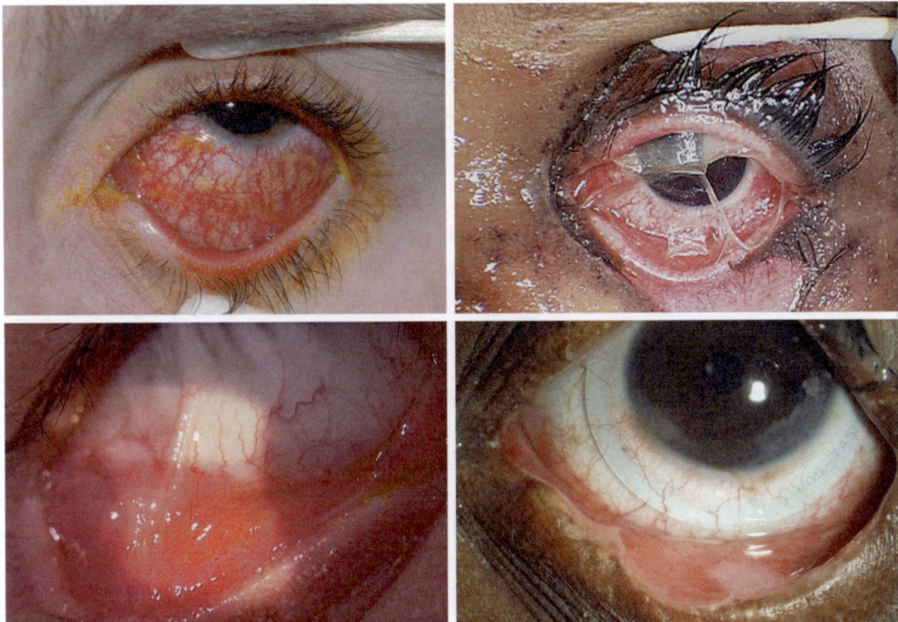

Fig. 7.1 Ocular manifestations of Stevens-Johnson syndrome and toxic epidermal necrolysis. Top left: bulbar conjunctival ulceration; Top right: desquamation of the ocular surface and lid margin; Bottom left: symblepharon; and Bottom right: lid margin and conjunctival keratinization, with a prosthetic replacement of the ocular surface ecosystem (PROSE device; Boston Foundation for Sight, Needham, Massachusetts, USA) in place. Illustration with permission from Catt CJ, Hamilton GM, Fish J, et al. Ocular Manifestations of Stevens-Johnson Syndrome and Toxic Epidermal Necrolysis in Children. Am J Ophthalmol 2016; 166:68–75

patients developed symblepharon, and 11% had ankyloblepharon. During the fifth and sixth weeks, 6–8% of patients had anterior blepharitis, trichiasis, and punctal occlusion. Between the third and fourth months, 22–25% of patients had chronic lid changes, including lid margin keratinization and meibomian gland dysfunction. Dry eye-related keratopathy and LSCD presented between 5 and 11 months. These findings occurred in the setting of acute phase treatment, where topical lubricants and steroids were used in 69% and 50% of children, respectively. Three patients with severe ocular involvement during the acute phase underwent amniotic membrane transplantation (AMT), and four patients had prosthetic replacement of the ocular surface ecosystem (PROSE) [28]. Without treatment, outcomes would likely have been worse. This is consistent with the authors' unpublished data that pediatric ocular disease is significantly more severe in the chronic phase when compared to adult patients. There are few natural history studies on SJS/TEN but studies on SJS/TEN where access to acute care is often poor appear to demonstrate significantly more severe chronic disease and pathology that includes corneal blindness when compared to regions where access to care is more robust [30, 31].

There are likely several factors that influence the evaluation and outcomes of SJS/TEN in the pediatric population. Oftentimes patients are intubated and sedated after admission for SJS/TEN. In these cases, full examination is possible at the bedside. If not, however, it can be very difficult to examine pediatric patients who are afraid, in pain, and do not understand the ramifications of undetected pathology. Because so much of acute ocular care is dependent on accurate examination, missed findings in this population can result in suboptimal treatment. Furthermore, treatment for moderate to severe ocular involvement involves the placement of an amniotic membrane on the ocular surface, which is unlikely to be tolerated by most pediatric patients. The traditional method for performing AMT often requires taking the patient to the operating room. Newer methods can be performed more easily at the bedside and can be done under sedation at the bedside. AMT is described in detail below.

After discharge from the hospital, evaluation of pediatric patients becomes even more difficult as the option for anesthesia and sedation is not immediately available. It is in the acute phase post-discharge, where most complications in this population occur (personal communication, HNS), likely due to a combination of examination difficulty, prolonged and more robust inflammation, and difficulty with treatment compliance. Treatment with specialty lenses such as PROSE is often required in the subacute phase. Though PROSE treatment is possible in the pediatric population, it is difficult and has higher rates of failure compared to adults [32]. The only long-term alternative to PROSE to protect the ocular surface is mucous membrane grafting (MMG) of the eyelids; however, this procedure often cannot be done in the subacute phase as the oral mucosa necessary for harvesting tissue is still healing from the acute SJS/TEN episode. This leaves the pediatric eye vulnerable to continued damage until MMG can be performed.

The largest to date series evaluating the chronic ocular sequalae of SJS/TEN was conducted by Basu and colleagues [30] and included 284 children with a median follow-up of 33 months. They compared eyes that were managed conservatively (topical artificial tears ± topical steroids, electrolysis, and punctal plugs) to those that had more definitive treatment either in the form of mucous membrane grafting (MMG), prosthetic replacement of the ocular surface ecosystem (PROSE), allogenic simple limbal epithelial transplantation (allo-SLET), or keratoprosthesis. They also classified eyes into 4 groups according to the degree of keratopathy: no keratopathy (NK), non-lid-related keratopathy (NLRK), lid-related keratopathy (LRK), and end-stage keratopathy (ESK). At the 5-year follow-up period, best corrected visual acuity (BCVA) was significantly improved with less progression of keratopathy in the definitive treatment group compared to the conservative treatment group. In the conservative treatment group, BCVA declined significantly in the NK (from 20/20 to 20/50), NLRK (from 20/40 to 20/320), and LRK (from 20/100 to 20/320) groups over 10 years. In the LRK group, MMG was more effective than PROSE, while a combination of both yielded the best results. The ocular and visual morbidity was significantly worse in patients ≤8 years. Please see Fig. 7.2 for a treatment algorithm proposed by Basu and colleagues for management of chronic ocular sequelae of SJS in children [30].

LSCD is a major cause of visual morbidity in SJS/TEN patients in the long term because of the inability of limbal stem cells to regenerate, the inability to perform

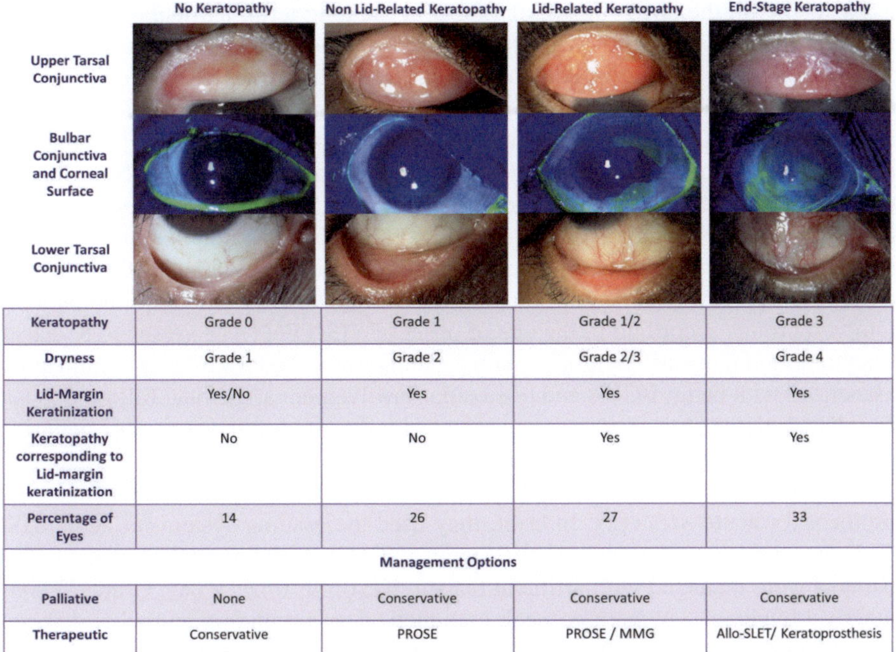

	No Keratopathy	Non Lid-Related Keratopathy	Lid-Related Keratopathy	End-Stage Keratopathy
Keratopathy	Grade 0	Grade 1	Grade 1/2	Grade 3
Dryness	Grade 1	Grade 2	Grade 2/3	Grade 4
Lid-Margin Keratinization	Yes/No	Yes	Yes	Yes
Keratopathy corresponding to Lid-margin keratinization	No	No	Yes	Yes
Percentage of Eyes	14	26	27	33
Management Options				
Palliative	None	Conservative	Conservative	Conservative
Therapeutic	Conservative	PROSE	PROSE / MMG	Allo-SLET/ Keratoprosthesis

Fig. 7.2 Overall management algorithm in eyes of children with chronic sequelae of Stevens-Johnson syndrome (SJS). This figure describes the general scheme of categorizing eyes into different therapeutic groups based on severity of keratopathy, degree of dryness, eyelid findings, and correlation between eyelid and corneal changes. Illustration with permission from Basu S, Shanbhag SS, Gokani A, et al. Chronic Ocular Sequelae of Stevens-Johnson Syndrome in Children: Long-term Impact of Appropriate Therapy on Natural History of Disease. Am J Ophthalmol 2018;189:17–28

autologous limbal stem cell transplantation (LSCT), and the poor outcomes of allogenic LSCT in SJS/TEN patients [24, 33]. Few studies have evaluated the success of LSCT in children with SJS/TEN. In the study by Basu and colleagues, 9 eyes underwent allo-SLET with improved BCVA from hand motions to 20/320 with a median follow-up of 15 months ($p < 0.0001$) [30]. This is a promising technique for LSCT but needs to be evaluated in larger studies. LSCT has notoriously poor outcomes in SJS/TEN patients [21]. A retrospective study by Choi and colleagues [29] evaluated the incidence and factors associated with LSCD development in children with SJS/TEN in the long term. The study included 19 SJS/TEN children, 6 of whom (32%) developed LSCD at a median of 3.5 months (mean 12.3 ± 21.3 months) after the onset of the disease. At the final follow-up visit, the logMAR BCVA was significantly better in patients without LSCD (0.05 ± 0.09) compared to those with LSCD (1.33 ± 1.52) ($p = 0.0055$). All patients without LSCD had BCVA $\geq 20/40$; however, in eyes with LSCD, 40% of eyes had a BCVA of <20/200. Three of six LSCD patients underwent combined penetrating keratoplasty and limbal allograft. All three patients had a postoperative graft infection, and graft failure developed in 2 patients. The severity of acute systemic manifestations was significantly associated with the development of LSCD in the long term, particularly liver dysfunction and C-reactive protein elevation; however, there was no significant association between the severity of acute ophthalmic manifestations and development of chronic ophthalmic complications including LSCD. Other studies, however, have shown a correlation between acute and chronic disease severity [34, 35]. There was no significant association between the systemic management of SJS/TEN during the acute phase of the disease and the development of LSCD [29]. Another retrospective case series conducted by Kim and colleagues [36] evaluated the effect of early treatment with systemic steroids or intravenous immunoglobulin (IVIG) or ocular treatment with AMT on ocular outcomes in SJS/TEN. They classified the patients into two groups according to the age of onset of SJS/TEN (≤18 versus >18 years). They reported that early treatment with systemic steroids or IVIG was significantly associated with better BCVA and less ocular involvement at the final follow-up visit in adult patients; however, there was no significant difference in the pediatric population.

Shanbhag and colleagues [34] evaluated the long-term impact of a management protocol for acute SJS/TEN. In brief, they used the grading system for acute SJS/TEN proposed by Sotozono and colleagues [37]. Grade 0 (no ocular involvement) patients were managed with artificial tears at least four times a day. Grade 1 (conjunctival hyperemia without corneal, conjunctival, or lid margin epithelial defects) patients were managed with topical artificial tears hourly, topical antibiotic (moxifloxacin 0.5%) three times a day, topical steroids (prednisolone acetate 1%) every 4 h, and a topical steroid ointment to the eyelids (fluorometholone 0.1%) every 4 h. Grade 2 (epithelial defects involving conjunctiva, cornea, or lid margin *without* membranes) patients were managed as Grade 1 with the addition of amniotic membrane treatment. They proposed the use of ProKera when amniotic membrane sheets are not available, or only corneal and/or bulbar conjunctiva are affected. Grade 3 (epithelial defects involving the conjunctiva, cornea, or lid margin *with* membranes) patients were managed like Grade 2, but AMT was required (Fig. 7.3) [34]. They compared the long-term outcomes of SJS/TEN patients who were treated prior to (group 1) and after (group 2) the implementation of this treatment protocol in terms of the final BCVA and incidence of chronic ocular complications. They reported a significantly higher percentage of eyes (92%) achieving BCVA ≥20/40 at the final follow-up visit in group 2 compared to eyes in group 1 (33%). Chronic vision-threatening complications were significantly higher in group 1 (67%) compared to group 2 (17%), with most complications occurring within the first 2 years of disease onset. Although their study included some pediatric patients, most of the patients were adults with a mean age of 34.2 ± 19 years (range; 5–58 years) in group 1 and 29.1 ± 18.7 (range; 1.5–71) in group 2 at the onset of SJS/TEN [34].

AMT was first reported as a treatment for acute SJS/TEN in 2002 by John and colleagues [38]. There are several techniques for AMT. In the pediatric population, we recommend the technique described by Shanbhag et al. [35] as it reduces the need for general anesthesia and can be performed at the bedside with light sedation [39–41]. In summary, a single sheet of cryopreserved continuous amniotic membrane (Amniograft, Bio-Tissue, Doral, FL) measuring 5 × 10 cm is placed over the entire ocular surface. The amniotic membrane is then anchored to the eyelids with

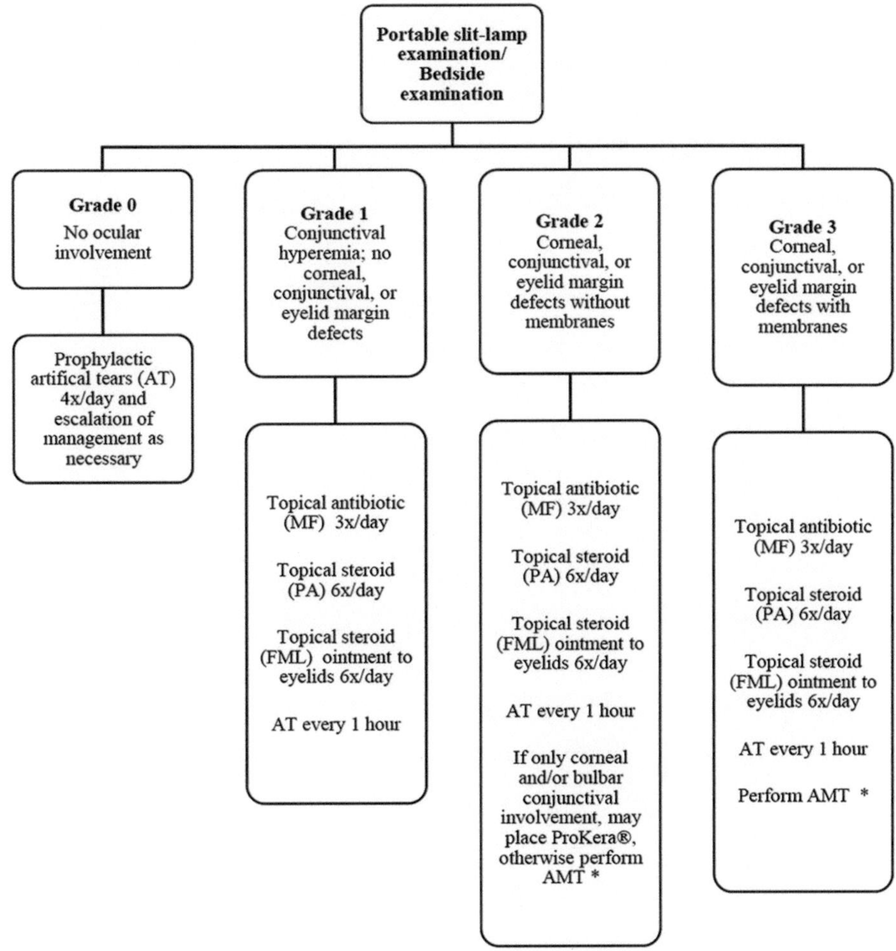

Fig. 7.3 Flow diagram outlining protocol for management of ocular manifestations in acute Stevens-Johnson syndrome/toxic epidermal necrolysis. (*MF* moxifloxacin 0.5%, *PA* prednisolone acetate 1%, *FML* fluorometholone 0.1%, *AT* artificial tears, *AMT* amniotic membrane transplantation).*Decision to perform AMT based on feasibility (intubation status, cooperation, etc.). ProKera is acceptable if only bulbar conjunctival or corneal involvement is present or when AMT is not feasible. Grade of acute involvement adapted from Sotozono's classification (Sotozono C, Ueta M, Nakatani E, et al. Predictive factors associated with acute ocular involvement in Stevens-Johnson syndrome and toxic epidermal necrolysis. Am J Ophthalmol 2015;160:228–37. e2). Illustration with permission from Shanbhag SS, Rashad R, Chodosh J, Saeed HN. Long-Term Effect of a Treatment Protocol for Acute Ocular Involvement in Stevens-Johnson Syndrome/Toxic Epidermal Necrolysis. Am J Ophthalmol 2019;208:331–41

cyanoacrylate glue 3–4 mm away from the lash line. After placing the amniotic membrane in the fornix, a symblepharon ring is inserted into the fornices to keep the amniotic membrane in place. The symblepharon ring is custom-made fashioned from intravenous tubing. A pre-made ring can also be used. See Fig. 7.4 for a detailed description.

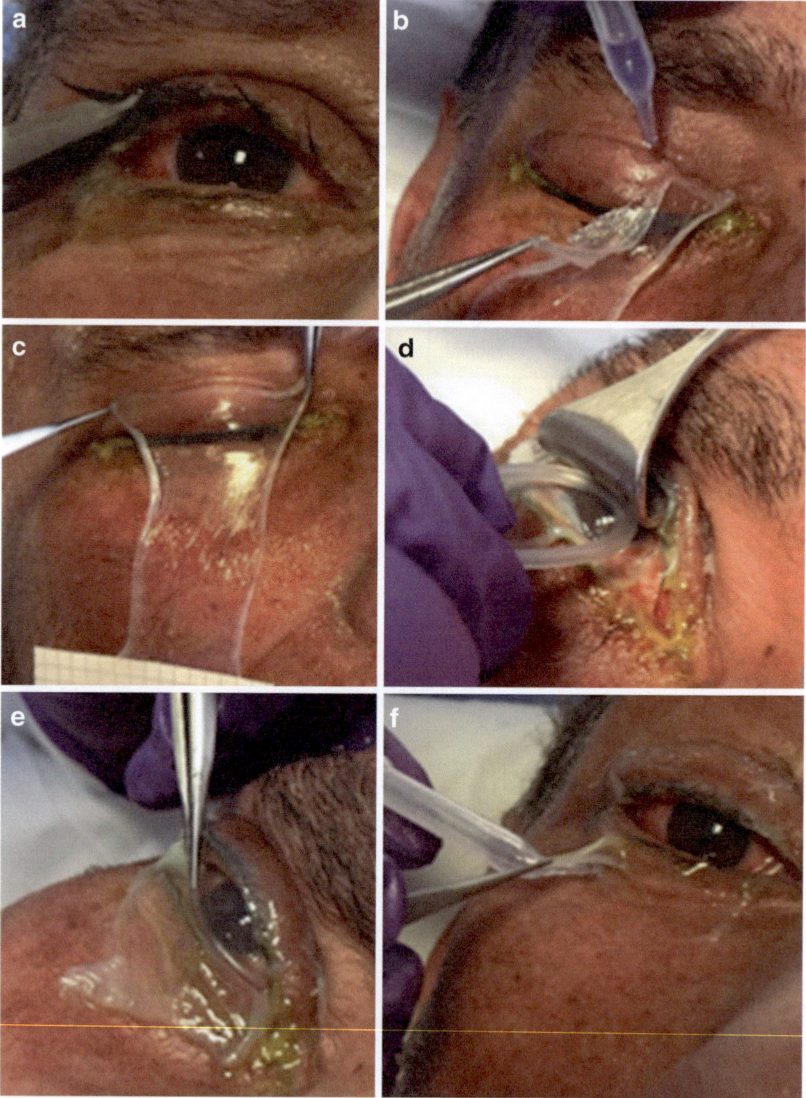

Fig. 7.4 Procedure for sutureless amniotic membrane transplantation (AMT) in the right eye of a patient with Stevens-Johnson syndrome with ocular surface and eyelid margin epithelial defects. (**a**) Upper and lower eyelashes are trimmed. (**b**) Cyanoacrylate glue is used to secure the amniotic membrane (AM) sheet (5 × 10 cm) to the upper eyelid. Care is taken to ensure glue is placed at least 4 mm above the eyelid margin. (**c**) AM is held across the upper eyelid for 30 s to ensure adhesion. (**d**) Desmarres lid retractor is used to retract the upper eyelid to allow the symblepharon ring to be placed in the superior fornix. (**e**) The symblepharon ring is then tucked into the inferior fornix. (**f**) The inferior margin of the AM is secured to the lower eyelid with cyanoacrylate glue. The patient should be able to close the eye without any lagophthalmos caused by the symblepharon ring. Illustration obtained with permission from Shanbhag SS, Chodosh J, Saeed HN. Sutureless amniotic membrane transplantation with cyanoacrylate glue for acute Stevens-Johnson syndrome/ toxic epidermal necrolysis. Ocul Surf. 2019;17(3):560–564

Mycoplasma Induced Rash and Mucositis

MIRM is a relatively newly identified entity in the literature that was first identified by Canavan and colleagues as being caused by *Mycoplasma pneumoniae* infection in 2015 [7, 42]. *M. pneumoniae* is a significant cause of community-acquired pneumonia (CAP) and responsible for 4–8% of all cases of bacterial CAP cases; however, it can cause a variety of extrapulmonary manifestations, including cardiac, vascular, gastrointestinal, dermatologic, and ophthalmic [43]. These manifestations can occur in the absence of pneumonia and have been proposed to occur by inducing local cytokine production, immune complex formation, or vascular occlusion [43]. See Fig. 7.5a–d for examples of clinical findings. Ocular involvement in MIRM is common in the acute phase, but long-term complications are often mild in contrast to SJS/TEN. Interestingly, the disease can be recurrent, which is

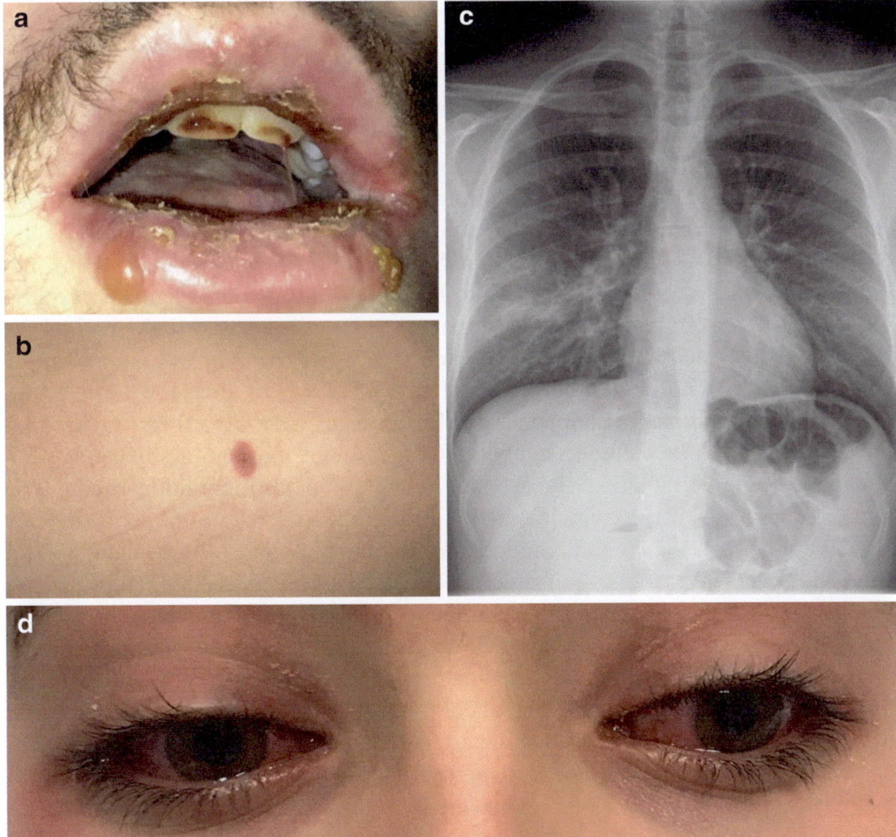

Fig. 7.5 Acute systemic and ocular manifestations of mycoplasma induced mucositis and rash including (**a**) mucositis and lip blisters, (**b**) target-like skin lesion, (**c**) chest X-ray showing right middle lobe pneumonia, (**d**) acute bilateral conjunctival hyperemia and erythematous periorbital skin

Table 7.1 Diagnostic criteria of classic, variant, and severe mycoplasma induced mucositis and rash (MIRM)

Diagnostic criteria	Classic	Sine rash	Severe
Cutaneous detachment	<10% BSA	<10% BSA	<10% BSA[a]
Number of mucosal sites involved	≥2[b]	≥2	≥2[b]
Lesions morphology	Few vesiculobullous lesions, or scattered atypical targets ± targetoid lesions	± few and fleeting morbilliform lesions, or few vesicles	Extensive widespread blisters or flat atypical targets

Evidence of atypical pneumonia
  1. Clinical: Fever, cough, positive auscultatory findings
  2. Laboratory: Increase in MP IgM antibodies, MP in oropharyngeal or bullae cultures or PCR, and/or serial cold agglutinins

BSA body surface area, *MP* mycoplasma pneumoniae, *PCR* polymerase chain reaction
[a]Rarely, it may involve >10% BSA
[b]Rarely, it may involve <2 mucosal sites

infrequently seen in SJS/TEN. A systematic review of 202 MIRM cases by Canavan and colleagues has largely established the ocular involvement of MIRM. They proposed four main differentiating points between MIRM and SJS/TEN [7]. MIRM is primarily a pediatric disease and predominantly affects multiple mucous membrane sites (usually ≥2). It also has variable and less impressive skin involvement (usually <10% TBSA) and a better prognosis than SJS/TEN [7]. They classified MIRM into 3 categories (classic, sine rash, and severe) according to four diagnostic criteria (Table 7.1). Canavan and colleagues reported the mean age of MIRM patients at the onset of the disease to be 11.9 ± 8.8 years. Sixty-six percent were male, which is also different than the demographics of SJS/TEN, where there is a female predominance [7]. Ocular involvement in MIRM ranges from 82–100% of cases [7, 44–46]. Ocular involvement is usually bilateral, with the most common ocular manifestations being conjunctival hyperemia, conjunctivitis, lid margin staining, meibomitis, ocular discharge, which may be purulent or mucoid, conjunctival and/or corneal epithelial defects, and conjunctival pseudomembranes. More than 90% of cases had complete resolution of mucocutaneous disease, including ocular disease [44–47]. Shah and colleagues [45] reported a series of five patients who presented at a mean age of 11.9 years. Ocular involvement was mild and without corneal involvement in all five cases. All five patients had conjunctivitis, including symblepharon formation. Two patients had conjunctival epithelial defects, and two had lid margin ulceration. The largest series to date of MIRM with ophthalmic involvement was reported by Gise and colleagues [44], which included 15 children, 13 (87%) of whom had ophthalmic involvement. Four patients had recurrent episodes ranging from 1 to 3 episodes, with the mean time of recurrence being 1.7 years. The mean age of patients at the initial episode was 10.9 years. They reported resolution of conjunctival symptoms at a mean of 12.1 days, while corneal symptoms resolved at a mean of 15.5 days. All 13 patients were treated with a topical steroid/antibiotic combination. AMT was performed in three patients, and one patient had ProKera placement. At the last follow-up, two patients had eyelid scarring, and one patient had mild symblepharon near the lateral canthus. 11 of 15 patients received oral or intravenous steroids, and nine patients received systemic antibiotic therapy. Another series by Rashad and colleagues [46] included 11 patients (6 patients were ≤ 18 years) with a mean age of 22.2 ± 15.2 at disease onset. The most common manifestation was conjunctival hyperemia, followed by meibomitis. None of the 11 patients required AMT, and all of them achieved a BCVA of 20/20 at the last follow-up visit. Three patients had long-term follow-up; two patients had distichiasis and/or trichiasis. Lastly, in a case series by Khalili and colleagues [47] including 10 MIRM patients, five patients had progressive ocular involvement during hospitalization, including a corneal epithelial defect in one patient and a new conjunctival epithelial defect in three patients. This highlights the need for close monitoring of these patients, despite the largely mild disease.

On literature review, 11 articles reported on the ocular manifestations of MIRM in the pediatric population, and the mean resolution time for conjunctival and corneal manifestations was 10.8 ± 2.2 days compared to 14.7 ± 2.6 days in adult MIRM; however, the difference was not statistically significant.

There is no consensus on the treatment of MIRM. Management of MIRM with ocular involvement includes systemic and ocular treatments [44–47]. Systemic treatment includes antibiotics, systemic steroids, IVIG, or plasmapheresis. Ocular treatment includes topical steroids, topical antibiotics, artificial tears, ProKera placement, or AMT. *M. pneumoniae* is protected by a cell membrane but lacks a cell wall; therefore, antibiotics that target the cell wall are unsuitable. Antibiotics that act by affecting cell metabolism and protein synthesis, such as macrolides, are more suitable for MIRM. Canavan and colleagues reported that out of 202 MIRM cases, 80% were managed by antibiotics (systemic or topical), 35% were managed by systemic steroids, and 8% by IVIG. One patient underwent plasmapheresis [7]. Several topical antibiotics have been used for the ocular management of MIRM, including tobramycin, gentamycin, erythromycin, moxifloxacin, and chloramphenicol, but it is unclear which treatments, if any, are superior.

Gise and colleagues [44] proposed a stepwise approach for management. All MIRM patients, even those without ocular involvement, were started on topical artificial tears with close follow-up. If there was lid margin (<1/3) and/or conjunctival involvement but no corneal involvement, they added topical antibiotic/steroid drops and ointment. More severe disease indicated by the presence of a corneal epithelial defect, conjunctival epithelial defect >1 cm, or lid margin staining affecting >1/3 of the margin were treated with AMT or a ProKera device [44].

Long-term ocular sequelae after MIRM are rare, and though there are no head-to-head studies, both acute and chronic complications are much less severe than in SJS/TEN [46].

Reactive/Recurrent Infectious Mucocutaneous Eruptions

Several recent reports have described a MIRM-like illness caused by infectious agents other than *M. pneumoniae*. Several infectious agents have been implicated in this illness, including adenovirus, influenza A virus, severe acute respiratory syndrome coronavirus 2 (SARS-CoV-2), rhinovirus, chlamydia, and streptococcus [48]. Ramien and Goldman [48] proposed a revised classification for pediatric blistering mucocutaneous conditions into two main categories: drug-induced epidermal necrolysis (DEN), including SJS/TEN, and RIME. RIME is considered to be an umbrella category including both MIRM and MIRM-like illnesses caused by infectious agents other than *M pneumoniae*. The rationale for their revised classification is the different management of the two categories, where treatment of DEN is based mainly on discontinuation of the triggering medication with early consideration of systemic immunotherapy, while treatment of RIME is focused on the identification and treatment of the infectious etiology and supportive therapy with or without immunosuppressive therapy [48]. There is no consensus on this, however, as many SJS/TEN cases are attributed to infectious causes as well.

The ophthalmic literature in RIME is very limited. Gise and colleagues [49] reported a series of 2 patients presenting with lid margin staining, mucoid discharge with matting of lashes, conjunctival hyperemia, and subconjunctival hemorrhage. The implicated agents were influenza A in one patient and adenovirus in the other patient. One patient had mild ocular involvement that was managed by topical artificial tears and topical steroids. The second patient had more severe involvement, which was treated with AMT; however, the outcome in both patients was excellent, with no chronic ocular sequalae.

As with MIRM, chronic ocular outcomes in RIME appear to be significantly less severe than that of SJS/TEN, but there are very limited data from which to draw definitive conclusions.

Summary

SJS/TEN, MIRM, and RIME are all mucocutaneous disorders that can affect the ocular surface in pediatric patients. Each is distinct with its unique ocular manifestations, course, prognosis, and complications. While ocular involvement in SJS/TEN is significantly more severe than in MIRM or RIME, all three require close monitoring and prophylactic treatment in the acute phase to prevent severe complications. Monitoring in the chronic phase appears to be more critical in SJS/TEN than MIRM or RIME, as severe vision-threatening disease is common in the former. However, the current literature is limited, and further studies are needed to fully understand the pathophysiology of disease and its visual implications, especially in the pediatric population.Acknowledgments and Disclosures*Funding*: None.

Financial disclosures: Dr. Elhusseiny, Dr. ElSheikh, and Dr. Saeed have no relevant financial disclosures.
Authorship: All authors attest that they meet the current ICMJE criteria for authorship.
Acknowledgments: None.

References

1. White KD, Abe R, Ardern-Jones M, et al. SJS/TEN 2017: building multidisciplinary networks to drive science and translation. The journal of allergy and clinical immunology. In Pract. 2018;6(1):38–69.
2. Kohanim S, Palioura S, Saeed HN, et al. Stevens-Johnson syndrome/toxic epidermal necrolysis – a comprehensive review and guide to therapy. I Systemic Disease. Ocul Surf. 2016;14(1):2–19.
3. Bastuji-Garin S, Rzany B, Stern RS, et al. Clinical classification of cases of toxic epidermal necrolysis, Stevens-Johnson syndrome, and erythema multiforme. Arch Dermatol. 1993;129(1):92–6.
4. Schalock PC, Dinulos JG, Pace N, et al. Erythema multiforme due to mycoplasma pneumoniae infection in two children. Pediatr Dermatol. 2006;23(6):546–55.
5. Hillebrand-Haverkort ME, Budding AE, bij de Vaate LA, van Agtmael MA. Mycoplasma pneumoniae infection with incomplete Stevens-Johnson syndrome. Lancet Infect Dis. 2008;8(10):586–7.
6. Tay YK, Huff JC, Weston WL. Mycoplasma pneumoniae infection is associated with Stevens-Johnson syndrome, not erythema multiforme (von Hebra). J Am Acad Dermatol. 1996;35(5 Pt 1):757–60.
7. Canavan TN, Mathes EF, Frieden I, Shinkai K. Mycoplasma pneumoniae-induced rash and mucositis as a syndrome distinct from Stevens-Johnson syndrome and erythema multiforme: a systematic review. J Am Acad Dermatol. 2015;72(2):239–45.
8. Meyer Sauteur PM, Seiler M, Trück J, et al. Diagnosis of mycoplasma pneumoniae pneumonia with measurement of specific antibody-secreting cells. Am J Respir Crit Care Med. 2019;200(8):1066–9.
9. Mazori DR, Nagarajan S, Glick SA. Recurrent reactive infectious mucocutaneous eruption (RIME): insights from a child with three episodes. Pediatr Dermatol. 2020;37(3):545–7.
10. Chan HL, Stern RS, Arndt KA, et al. The incidence of erythema multiforme, Stevens-Johnson syndrome, and toxic epidermal necrolysis. A population-based study with particular reference to reactions caused by drugs among outpatients. Arch Dermatol. 1990;126(1):43–7.
11. Roujeau JC, Stern RS. Severe adverse cutaneous reactions to drugs. N Engl J Med. 1994;331(19):1272–85.
12. Prendiville JS, Hebert AA, Greenwald MJ, Esterly NB. Management of Stevens-Johnson syndrome and toxic epidermal necrolysis in children. J Pediatr. 1989;115(6):881–7.
13. Sheridan RL, Weber JM, Schulz JT, et al. Management of severe toxic epidermal necrolysis in children. J Burn Care Rehabil. 1999;20(6):497–500.
14. Koh MJ, Tay YK. Stevens-Johnson syndrome and toxic epidermal necrolysis in Asian children. J Am Acad Dermatol. 2010;62(1):54–60.
15. Chatproedprai S, Wutticharoenwong V, Tempark T, Wananukul S. Clinical features and treatment outcomes among children with Stevens-Johnson syndrome and toxic epidermal necrolysis: a 20-year study in a tertiary referral hospital. Dermatol Res Pract. 2018;2018:3061084.
16. Quirke KP, Beck A, Gamelli RL, Mosier MJ. A 15-year review of pediatric toxic epidermal necrolysis. J Burn Care Res. 2015;36(1):130–6.
17. Dibek Misirlioglu E, Guvenir H, Bahceci S, et al. Severe cutaneous adverse drug reactions in pediatric patients: a multicenter study. J Allergy Clin Immunol Pract. 2017;5(3):757–63.

18. Finkelstein Y, Soon GS, Acuna P, et al. Recurrence and outcomes of Stevens-Johnson syndrome and toxic epidermal necrolysis in children. Pediatrics. 2011;128(4):723–8.
19. Levi N, Bastuji-Garin S, Mockenhaupt M, et al. Medications as risk factors of Stevens-Johnson syndrome and toxic epidermal necrolysis in children: a pooled analysis. Pediatrics. 2009;123(2):e297–304.
20. Singh S, Jakati S, Shanbhag SS, et al. Lid margin keratinization in Stevens-Johnson syndrome: review of pathophysiology and histopathology. Ocul Surf. 2021;21:299–305.
21. Kohanim S, Palioura S, Saeed HN, et al. Acute and chronic ophthalmic involvement in Stevens-Johnson syndrome/toxic epidermal necrolysis – a comprehensive review and guide to therapy. II Ophthalmic Disease. Ocul Surf. 2016;14(2):168–88.
22. Ibrahim OMA, Yagi-Yaguchi Y, Noma H, et al. Corneal higher-order aberrations in Stevens-Johnson syndrome and toxic epidermal necrolysis. Ocul Surf. 2019;17(4):722–8.
23. Rashad R, Shanbhag SS, Kwan J, et al. Chronic ocular complications in lamotrigine vs. trimethoprim-sulfamethoxazole induced Stevens-Johnson syndrome/toxic epidermal necrolysis. Ocul Surf. 2021;21:16–8.
24. Wall V, Yen MT, Yang M-C, et al. Management of the Late Ocular Sequelae of Stevens-Johnson syndrome. Ocul Surf. 2003;1(4):192–201.
25. Yip LW, Thong BY, Lim J, et al. Ocular manifestations and complications of Stevens-Johnson syndrome and toxic epidermal necrolysis: an Asian series. Allergy. 2007;62(5):527–31.
26. Morales ME, Purdue GF, Verity SM, et al. Ophthalmic manifestations of Stevens-Johnson syndrome and toxic epidermal necrolysis and relation to SCORTEN. Am J Ophthalmol. 2010;150(4):505–10.e1.
27. Jones WG, Halebian P, Madden M, et al. Drug-induced toxic epidermal necrolysis in children. J Pediatr Surg. 1989;24(2):167–70.
28. Catt CJ, Hamilton GM, Fish J, et al. Ocular manifestations of Stevens-Johnson syndrome and toxic epidermal necrolysis in children. Am J Ophthalmol. 2016;166:68–75.
29. Choi SH, Kim MK, Oh JY. Corneal Limbal stem cell deficiency in children with Stevens-Johnson syndrome. Am J Ophthalmol. 2019;199:1–8.
30. Basu S, Shanbhag SS, Gokani A, et al. Chronic ocular sequelae of Stevens-Johnson syndrome in children: long-term impact of appropriate therapy on natural history of disease. Am J Ophthalmol. 2018;189:17–28.
31. Shanbhag SS, Shah S, Singh M, et al. Lid-related keratopathy in Stevens-Johnson syndrome: natural course and impact of therapeutic interventions in children and adults. Am J Ophthalmol. 2020;219:357–65.
32. Wang Y, Rao R, Jacobs DS, Saeed HN. Prosthetic replacement of the ocular surface ecosystem treatment for ocular surface disease in pediatric patients with Stevens-Johnson syndrome. Am J Ophthalmol. 2019;201:1–8.
33. Elhusseiny AM, Soleimani M, Eleiwa TK, et al. Current and emerging therapies for Limbal stem cell deficiency. Stem Cells Transl Med. 2022;11(3):259–68.
34. Shanbhag SS, Rashad R, Chodosh J, Saeed HN. Long-term effect of a treatment protocol for acute ocular involvement in Stevens-Johnson syndrome/toxic epidermal necrolysis. Am J Ophthalmol. 2019;208:331–41.
35. Shanbhag SS, Chodosh J, Saeed HN. Sutureless amniotic membrane transplantation with cyanoacrylate glue for acute Stevens-Johnson syndrome/toxic epidermal necrolysis. Ocul Surf. 2019;17(3):560–4.
36. Kim KH, Park SW, Kim MK, Wee WR. Effect of age and early intervention with a systemic steroid, intravenous immunoglobulin or amniotic membrane transplantation on the ocular outcomes of patients with Stevens-Johnson syndrome. Korean J Ophthalmol. 2013;27(5):331–40.
37. Sotozono C, Ueta M, Nakatani E, et al. Predictive factors associated with acute ocular involvement in Stevens-Johnson syndrome and toxic epidermal necrolysis. Am J Ophthalmol. 2015;160(2):228–37.e2.
38. John T, Foulks GN, John ME, et al. Amniotic membrane in the surgical management of acute toxic epidermal necrolysis. Ophthalmology. 2002;109(2):351–60.

39. Ma KN, Thanos A, Chodosh J, et al. A novel technique for amniotic membrane transplantation in patients with acute Stevens-Johnson syndrome. Ocul Surf. 2016;14(1):31–6.
40. Saeed HN, Chodosh J. Ocular manifestations of Stevens-Johnson syndrome and their management. Curr Opin Ophthalmol. 2016;27(6):522–9.
41. Elhusseiny AM, Gise R, Scelfo C, Mantagos IS. Amniotic membrane transplantation in a 2-month-old infant with toxic epidermal necrolysis. Am J Ophthalmol Case Rep. 2021;21:101017.
42. Mayor-Ibarguren A, Feito-Rodriguez M, González-Ramos J, et al. Mucositis secondary to chlamydia pneumoniae infection: expanding the mycoplasma pneumoniae-induced rash and Mucositis concept. Pediatr Dermatol. 2017;34(4):465–72.
43. Narita M. Pathogenesis of extrapulmonary manifestations of mycoplasma pneumoniae infection with special reference to pneumonia. J Infect Chemother. 2010;16(3):162–9.
44. Gise R, Elhusseiny AM, Scelfo C, Mantagos IS. Mycoplasma Pneumoniae-induced rash and Mucositis: a longitudinal perspective and proposed management criteria. Am J Ophthalmol. 2020;219:351–6.
45. Shah PR, Williams AM, Pihlblad MS, Nischal KK. Ophthalmic manifestations of mycoplasma-induced rash and Mucositis. Cornea. 2019;38(10):1305–8.
46. Rashad R, Elhusseiny AM, Shanbhag SS, et al. Acute ophthalmic manifestations in mycoplasma induced rash and mucositis. Ocul Surf. 2022;24:145–7.
47. Khalili A, Ackerman IM, Gorski MG, et al. Ophthalmic findings of Mycoplasma–Induced Rash And Mucositis (MIRM) distinct from Stevens-Johnson syndrome. J AAPOS. 2021;25(6):348.e1–6.
48. Ramien M, Goldman JL. Pediatric SJS-TEN: Where are we now? F1000Res. 2020;9:F1000. Faculty Rev-982
49. Gise R, Elhusseiny AM, Scelfo C, Mantagos IS. Ocular involvement in recurrent infectious mucocutaneous eruption (RIME): a variation on a theme. J AAPOS. 2021;25(1):62–4.

Chapter 8
Pediatric Neurotrophic Keratopathy

Piseth Dalin Chea, Dorian Ariel Zeidenweber, and Simon S. M. Fung

Introduction

Definition

Neurotrophic keratopathy (NK) is often defined as a degenerative condition of the cornea characterized by an absence of cornea sensitivity and impairment of epithelial healing [1]. However, as we detail later in this chapter, many of the possible causes of NK in the pediatric population are not due to a degenerative condition, and therefore the above definition does not adequately address these cases. The proposed definition by Dua et al. may be more suitable [2], who stated that "neurotrophic keratopathy is a disease related to alterations in corneal nerves leading to impairment in sensory and trophic function with consequent breakdown of the corneal epithelium, affecting health and integrity of the tear film, epithelium and stroma." The lack of cornea surface sensory innervation is the risk factor of tear film instability, epitheliopathy, progression to stromal lysis or melting, and subsequently perforation if not managed appropriately and timely.

P. D. Chea
Cornea and External Diseases, Jules Stein Eye Institute, University of California,
Los Angeles, CA, USA

Calmette Hospital, Phnom Penh, Cambodia

D. A. Zeidenweber
Cornea and External Diseases, Jules Stein Eye Institute, University of California,
Los Angeles, CA, USA

S. S. M. Fung (✉)
Pediatric Ophthalmology, Cornea and External Diseases, Jules Stein Eye Institute, University
of California, Los Angeles, CA, USA
e-mail: simonfung@mednet.ucla.edu

© The Author(s), under exclusive license to Springer Nature
Switzerland AG 2023
A. Traish, V. P. Douglas (eds.), *Pediatric Ocular Surface Disease*,
https://doi.org/10.1007/978-3-031-30562-7_8

Epidemiology

Neurotrophic keratopathy is a rare disease with limited epidemiologic data. NK is considered as a rare/orphan disease (ORPHA13756) affecting 1.6–5 per 10,000 individuals [2–4]. This figure is mostly extrapolated from the prevalence of conditions that are associated with neurotrophic keratopathy, including herpetic keratitis (149/100,000) [5], 12.8% of herpes zoster keratitis (26/100,000) [6], and neurotrauma after trigeminal neuralgia procedure (0.02/10,000) [7]. However, the prevalence of NK is likely to be under reported, with data from tertiary referral centers reporting disease prevalence between (9–22/10,000) [8, 9]. It is noteworthy that much of the epidemiologic data were derived from more economically developed countries, and there is a paucity of data regarding NK in less developed countries, even though it may be more prevalent due to higher incidences of cornea infection and ocular chemical injuries. Information on the epidemiology of pediatric NK is even more scarce. In a clinical study by Bonini and colleagues, 13.9% had the onset of NK before the age of 6 years old among the 43 patients; all of them were female even though the overall cohort did not demonstrate any gender predilection [10, 11].

Cornea Nerve Structure and Function

Cornea has the richest innervation compared to other parts of human body; 300–600 times more sensitive than skin with a central corneal nerve density of approximately 7000 nociceptors per square millimeter [12, 13]. Innervation of cornea epithelium first occurs at 5 months of gestation [14]. Cornea sensory nerves originate from the ophthalmic division of trigeminal ganglion; the nerve bundles lose their perineurium and myelin sheaths at 1 mm after entering the corneal limbus. Surrounded by Schwann cells, these nerves travel anteriorly within the anterior corneal stroma to form a sub-epithelial nerve plexus between anterior stroma and Bowman layer [15]. The nerve fiber then penetrates through Bowman layer to form the subbasal nerve plexus (SBNP) between Bowman's layer and basal epithelium. The SBNP gives rise to superficial nerve branches that ascend perpendicularly and terminating in the cornea epithelium [16].

The corneal nerves have two vital roles in the maintenance of a healthy ocular surface: protective reflexes and trophic factors secretion. Reaction to noxious stimuli or injuries on the corneal surface triggers the protective reflexes (e.g., blinking) and neuro-secretory reflexes (e.g., tearing) [17]. Corneal innervation also provides nutrient and trophic factors in the maintenance of the anatomical integrity, clarity, and function of the corneal epithelial surface [18]. Cornea nerves releases many epitheliotropic neuromediators including substance P (SP), neurokinin A, calcitonin gene-related peptide (CGRP), acetylcholine, cholecystokinin, galanin, noradrenaline, serotonin, neuropeptide Y (NYP), vasoactive intestinal peptide (VIP), neurotensin, and beta endorphin [11, 19]. Conversely, cornea epithelial cells and corneal

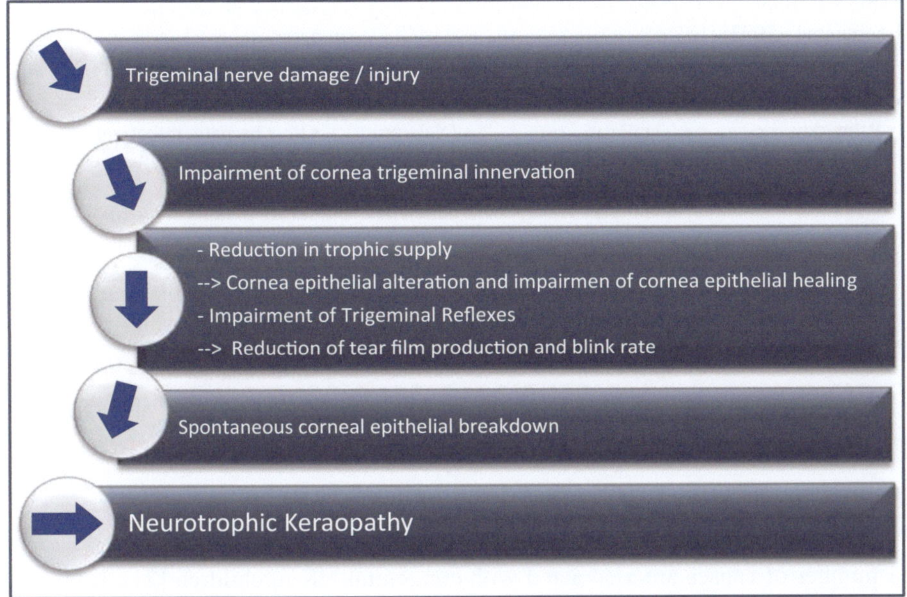

Fig. 8.1 Role of cornea trigeminal innervation in neurotrophic keratitis. Adapted from Mastropasua et al. (2017) [20]

keratocytes play an important role in nerve fibers survival, differentiation, and maturation by releasing nerve growth factors (NFG), neurotrophins, and neuropeptides. Insults to any portion of the pathway of innervation negatively affects the delicate homeostasis, reducing trophic supply to corneal epithelial cells, impairing cornea wound healing and tear film function, and ultimately contributing to ocular surface instability that is characteristic of NK (Fig. 8.1) [20].

Etiology of NK

Any disruptions along the pathway of corneal innervation can result in NK, with potential causes include ocular and central nervous system lesion or injuries, genetic conditions, and systemic diseases affecting different levels of the fifth cranial nerve. The most frequent ocular cause of corneal nerve damage in adult is keratitis secondary to herpes simplex and herpes zoster infections. Another common cause in adults is trauma or surgery to the cornea or the ocular surface, including thermal or chemical burn, anterior segment surgery (e.g., cornea transplantation and laser ablative procedures), and chronic contact lens wear [1]. In children, congenital and iatrogenic causes of NK are more commonly encountered in the pediatric cohort, as listed in Table 8.1 [10]. The following section will discuss a selected number of conditions that are more commonly encountered in children.

Table 8.1 Etiology of cornea sensory impairment leading to neurotrophic keratitis. Adapted from Bonini et al. (2003) [10]

Genetic	CNS	Systemic disease	Ocular
• Riley-day syndrome • Goldenhar-Gorlin syndrome • Mobius syndrome • Familial corneal hypoesthesia	• Neoplasm • Acoustic neuroma • Trigeminal neuralgia • Post neurosurgical procedures • Surgical injury to trigeminal nerve • Aneurysms • Stroke	• Diabetes • Leprosy • Vitamin A deficiency	• Post herpetic infections • Ocular surface injury (chemical or thermal burn) • Drug toxicity (topical anesthetics abuse and anti-glaucoma) • Post-surgical and laser ablation (cornea or perilimbal incision) • Chronic ocular surface inflammation • Chronic contact lens wear • Cornea dystrophy

Congenital Causes of Pediatric Neurotrophic Keratopathy

A number of causes are associated with congenital NK in children [21]. Ramaesh and colleagues proposed a classification system to categorize these diagnoses (Table 8.2). It is outside the scope of this review to describe all the possible diagnoses in detail, and therefore only the more commonly encountered conditions will be discussed here.

Isolated Congenital Cornea Anesthesia: Normally the onset of the disease manifests between 8 and 12 months. It is a challenging entity to diagnosed, requiring a high index of suspicion in the setting of recurrent painless epithelial defect [22, 23].

Familial Trigeminal Anesthesia: Characterized by reduced sensation in the area of trigeminal innervation. Only a few cases have been described in literature, and many did not differentiate between corneal hypoesthesia associated with other syndromes and isolated trigeminal anesthesia [22].

Möbius Syndrome: Characterized by non-progressive congenital paralysis of facial and abducens nerve. Clinical manifestations, inability to suck at birth, feeding swallowing and choking problems, strabismus, and lack of facial expression. Most cases are sporadic in nature with no family history or gender preference. Important to note is that the efferent facial nerve is most heavily involved, therefore the cornea damage is compounded by exposure keratopathy and co-existing NK. Other ophthalmologic abnormalities described include hypertelorism, epicanthus, and congenital ptosis [22].

Familial Dysautonomia (Riley-Day Syndrome): This entity belongs to the family of hereditary sensory and autonomic neuropathies. With a prevalence of less than 1 in 1,000,000, familial dysautonomia is an autosomal recessive disorder that affects the development and sensory function of nerves throughout the body. Apart from

Table 8.2 New classification of congenital cornea anesthesia. Adapted from Ramaesh et al. (2007) [21]

Isolated corneal involvement
Familial
(a) Normal corneal nerves
(b) Reduced corneal nerves
Isolated
Associated with ocular conditions
(a) Contralateral anophthalmos and macrosomia
(b) Hereditary fleck corneal dystrophy
Decrease sensation in the distribution of the trigeminal nerve with no other neurological and systemic features
(a) Familial
(b) Sporadic
Associated with neurological disorders
(a) Mobius syndrome
(b) Riley-day syndrome
(c) Generalized insensitivity to pain and muscle weakness
(d) Vertebral and other congenital defects
(e) Cerebellar ataxia, cogwheel ocular pursuits, anal atresia, and abnormal optokinetic nystagmus
Congenital insensitivity to pain
Associated with somatic disorders
(a) MURCS (Mullerian duct and renal aplasia, cervical somite dysplasia)
(b) Goldenhar syndrome (OAVD- oculo-auriculo-vertebral dysplasia)
(c) Hypohidrotic ectodermal dysplasia
(d) VACTERL association (vertebral, anal, cardiovascular, tracheoesophageal, renal, and limb defects)

NK, it can also present in the eye as corneal ulceration secondary to severe dry eye from congenital alacrimia in up to 50% of affected individuals as well as swallowing problems, breath holding spells, and inability to feel pain and changes in temperature.

Oculo-Auriculo-Vertebral Spectrum (Goldenhar-Gorlin Syndrome): It is an uncommon congenital defect that affects the embryological structures derived from the first and second branchial arches. Only 1–2% of cases are transmitted with an autosomal dominant pattern, the rest are sporadic transmission. Clinical manifestations include craniofacial abnormalities involving the ears (microtia) and the face (hemifacial microsomia). It can also affect the heart and eyes (epibulbar dermoid) in 50% of patients.

Congenital Insensitivity to Pain with Anhidrosis (CIPA): This is an extremely rare condition with less than 100 cases reported in literature. Once there is damage to corneal sensory innervation, clinically we find epitheliopathy that progresses to recurrent epithelial defects that encounter hardship to heal. Progression of the disease with corneal ulceration, stromal melting, infection, perforation, and blindness can occur if left untreated [22].

Acquired Causes of Pediatric Neurotrophic Keratopathy

Acquired pediatric NK is often due to lesions in the cranial nerve system, with potential causes ranging from space occupying intracranial neoplasia, head trauma, or aneurysm and neurosurgery affecting the trigeminal nervous pathway [24–29]. Lambley et al. (2015) reported that posterior fossa tumors (30.8%), in particular ependymoma, were the most common cause of corneal anesthesia among 33 children in a Canadian tertiary pediatric center [30].

Impairment of corneal innervation can also be caused by several acquired systemic or local disorders. Examples in the pediatric population include viral infections such as herpetic eye disease, eye drop toxicity, and ocular surgery [9, 31]. However, systemic conditions such as diabetes or multiple sclerosis causing NK are rarely reported in pediatric population.

Viral infection: Herpes simplex (HSV) related keratitis is one of the most prevalent and visually morbid ocular infection both in the adult and pediatric population. The prevalence of HSV has been estimated to be up to 50–90% both in adult and pediatric population. Clinical manifestations of viral keratitis in children include tearing, eyelid swelling, decrease in visual acuity, and photophobia. However, up to two-thirds of children affected may not report any symptoms, resulting in delayed presentation [32, 33]. Furthermore, while the condition is characterized by epithelial dendritic keratitis, children often present with immune stromal keratitis, and recurrent disease is more common in the pediatric population, occurring in 38–80% of patients [32, 33], making the condition challenging to diagnose. However, it is believed that NK is less likely to be caused by prior herpetic infections as the latter require a long history of multiple recurrence to induce corneal nerve damage [22].

Varicella zoster infection in children usually present as vesicular rash (chickenpox). While herpes zoster ophthalmicus—a reactivation of virus in the trigeminal nerve innervation—is rare in non-immunocompromised children [34], it is nonetheless a potentially devastating condition that can result in interstitial keratitis, anterior uveitis, sclerokeratouveitis, and NK [35].

Bacterial infection: Bacterial keratitis is a major cause of corneal blindness in children in developing countries, with predisposing factors being ocular trauma (21%), ocular surface disease (17.7%), and vitamin A deficiency. Bacterial keratitis could be a rare cause of neurotrophic keratitis in the pediatric population [36].

Iatrogenic causes: Iatrogenic causes of pediatric NK can be categorized as either medical or surgical. Medical causes such as prolonged use and abuse of topical medications can lead to NK [31]. Prolonged contact lens wear can also be a cause of NK. However, the authors have not found them to be common etiologies in pediatric NK.

A number of surgical interventions have been reported to cause NK in the pediatric setting. These procedures include ophthalmic surgeries such as keratoplasties or corneal refractive surgery, although more commonly pediatric NK is associated with neurosurgical interventions involving or in the proximity of the trigeminal nervous pathway, resulting in corneal hypoesthesia and NK [31]. Furthermore, it is not an uncommon scenario in which both the trigeminal and the facial nerves are affected, resulting in a densely anesthetic cornea that is exposed due to concurrent lagophthalmos. Therefore, in children with ocular concerns and a history of neuro-surgical interventions, the authors advise careful assessment of corneal sensation to reveal any occult corneal hypoesthesia and previously undiagnosed NK.

Trauma: Ocular chemical injuries or burns can lead to permanent decrease in the sensitivity of the cornea and cause acquired NK. Ocular chemical injuries are common especially in developing countries, although it is unclear how many of these cases ultimately result in NK in children.

Corneal dystrophy: Although rare in the pediatric population, corneal dystrophies may cause NK in long term. The buildup of material in the corneal stroma can cause decrease in corneal sensitivity and as a result decrease blinking.

Systemic diseases: Diabetes mellitus and multiple sclerosis play a very limited role in the pediatric population. However, although uncommon in developed countries, nutritional deficiency is an important cause of pediatric NK. Over 100 million children worldwide are estimated to have vitamin A deficiency and over 5 million have ocular manifestations. This vision threatening disorder can lead to corneal blindness from neurotrophic keratopathy and severe keratomalacia [37]. Vitamin B12 deficiency may also be a cause of NK [38].

Diagnostic Approaches in Pediatric NK

Diagnosis of pediatric NK could be challenging and often rely on qualitative instead of quantitative assessments. A high index of suspicion and a careful examination, including corneal sensation assessment, is crucial in the diagnosis of NK in children. Clinical imaging such as Anterior Segment Optical Coherence Tomography (AS-OCT), In Vivo Confocal Microscopy (IVCM), and Magnetic Resonance Imaging (MRI) of the brain and the orbit may be useful in the evaluation of pediatric NK and guide its management, but these techniques may not be suitable in all pediatric cases.

Clinical History and Symptoms

Inherent to the fact that there is reduced corneal and ocular surface sensation, ocular discomfort is rarely reported by NK patients. This is particularly the case in children, who often could not or would not verbalize their symptoms. Collateral history therefore is of paramount importance. The parents accompanying the child suspicious of having NK may report mild but persistent conjunctival hyperemia. They may also report the phenomenon of oculo-digital reflex, in which the child is observed to vigorously rub or even press the ocular surface. Other clues may reside in the information from the referring physician, who may have observed a non-painful persistent epithelial defect or an infectious ulcerative lesion. Prior recurrent attendances to pediatric emergency department with cornea abrasion should also raise the suspicion of cornea anesthesia and NK [39]. History of neurosurgery, ocular or head trauma, use of topical and systemic medication, and congenital or systemic conditions are all relevant information that can point toward a diagnosis of pediatric NK [2].

Ocular Examination

In a child suspected of NK, a detailed cranial nerve examination is an important part of the patient assessment. Identification of cranial nerve impairments may help in confirming the diagnosis of NK, localizing the underlying neurological insult, and optimizing the therapeutic approach for the patient. For instance, a combined third, fourth, and sixth cranial nerve palsy with NK may prompt an evaluation for cavernous sinus pathologies; NK associated with seventh and eighth cranial nerve dysfunction may indicate a potential cause of acoustic neuroma. Note that in the presence of a seventh nerve palsy, the resultant lagophthalmos, tear production, and blink reflex impairment complicate the outlook of NK, and a permanent tarsorrhaphy should be strongly considered (see Sect. 8.5: Therapeutic options and challenges) [40].

A detailed slit lamp examination can provide information on the potential etiology as well as the severity of NK (see next section). Apart from corneal epitheliopathy, corneal stromal loss, scaring, or vascularization can be signs of reduced corneal sensation in children's eyes. Corneal stromal infiltration in the area of a persistent epithelial defect may indicate a superimposed infection in the area. The presence of iris defect or atrophy may be a sign of a previous herpetic infection.

The use of vital dyes such as fluorescein on the ocular surface can be instrumental in grading corneal and conjunctival abnormality, including the degree of punctate erosion and the presence and size of any corneal epithelial defects. The use of vital dye is particularly useful in toddlers and young children, who can be challenging to examine, and clinicians may only have brief moments to assess the child with a portable system or even at a distance.

NK-associated ocular surface dryness can be due to deceased tear production and tear film instability, which can be detected with Schirmer's test and tear break-up time (TBUT), although they may not be easy to perform in the very young children. Optic nerve pallor can be an indication of intracranial neoplasm [4].

Cornea Sensation

The assessment of the corneal sensation is crucial in the confirmation and the classification of NK severity in adult and in children alike. It is important to note that corneal and conjunctival sensitivity in young children including infants were not significantly different to that in adults, suggesting that sensory pathway is well developed at the time of birth [41], and therefore there is no lower age limits for corneal sensation testing.

A number of tests can be used to assess the corneal sensation, including the cotton wisp, Cochet-Bonnet esthesiometer, and Belmonte esthesiometer. The use of cotton wisp or folded tissue is often used as a quick and easy test in the office. By touching the corneal surface and observe for a response, it can only provide a qualitative assessment of the corneal nerve function. However, this is usually restricted to a binary (present/absent) result of the corneal nerve function. Cochet-Bonnet esthesiometer is a device consisting of a nylon filament of 0.08 or 0.12 mm in diameter, with a maximum length of 60 mm. By varying the length of the nylon filament, a different pressure would be generated when it is used to stimulate the corneal nerves by gently touching the corneal surface [42]. Once the patient reports a corneal touch, the length of filament at which the response could be read and could be recorded quantitatively [43]. In contrast, the Belmonte non-contact esthesiometer stimulates the corneal nerves by gaseous emissions produced at different temperatures, pressures, and concentration of CO_2. This has the advantage of being able to quantitatively assess the cornea sensitivity to different mechanical, chemical, and thermal stimuli separately [44]. However, the device is not commercially available and is mostly restricted to research purposes only.

In children, the method of corneal sensation testing can vary with age. A simple cornea sensation test can be the administration of eye drops that causes ocular irritation, such as hypertonic saline [45], or anticholinergic mydriatics. In our experience, however, we found the observation of the blink reflex after gentle corneal touch using a Cochet-Bonnet esthesiometer to be an easy and informative testing method. This allows even the very young to be tested and provides at least qualitative and often quantitative results. When a child can provide reliable response to cornea sensation test, the esthesiometer could be used to assess different areas of the cornea (central, nasal, inferior, temporal, and superior) to give further information of the distribution and function of corneal innervation.

During assessment of corneal sensation, it is useful to note that ocular surgeries may influence the findings. The pattern of sensory loss and speed of recovery depend on the type and extent of the procedure and presumably their effects on the corneal nerve fibers [46]. Table 8.3 summarizes the approximate recovery time of cornea sensation after various types of ocular procedures.

Table 8.3 Ocular surgery/procedure and recovery of corneal sensation

Procedure	Cornea sensation recovery period
Large-incision cataract surgery	1–2 years
Manual small-incision cataract surgery	3–9 months
Penetrating and anterior lamellar keratoplasty	2 years
Arcuate keratotomy	1 year
Tectonic overlay grafts and epikeratophakia	5–10 years
Intrastromal rings	1 year
Photorefractive keratectomy	<6 months
Phototherapeutic keratectomy	Increase cornea sensitivity
LASIK	>6 months
Collagen cross-linking	6–12 months
Strabismus surgery	2–4 Months
Retinal detachment surgery	>6 months

Special Investigation

In Vivo Confocal Microscopy (IVCM)

In vivo confocal microscopy is one of the most important devices in the evaluation of corneal innervation due to its ability to illustrate the subbasal nerve plexus and nerve characteristics including the nerve fiber density, length, tortuosity, angulation, thickness, reflectivity, and branching patterns [2, 47, 48]. In NK, IVCM can be helpful in the assessment and monitoring of pathological cornea nerve changes in NK patients (Fig. 8.2). It has been shown that in NK associated with pre-ganglionic and partial trigeminal ganglion lesions, IVCM may demonstrate a normal subbasal plexus, whereas NK associated with post-ganglionic or complete ganglionic lesions the subbasal plexus is attenuated or lost [49]. Study showed an association between

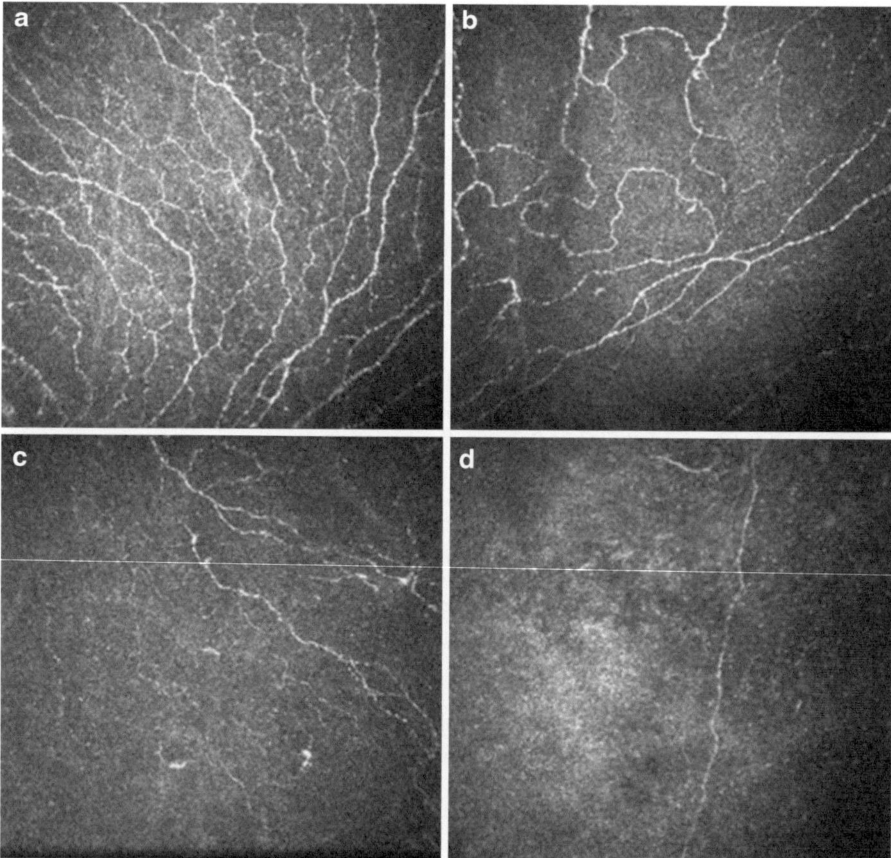

Fig. 8.2 Image of IVCM comparing (**a**) intact cornea subepithelial nerve plexus in healthy eye versus neurotrophic cornea with (**b**) mild, (**c**) moderate, or (**d**) severe reduction in nerve density and branching. (Image from Mastropasqua et al. (2017)) [20]

anesthetic cornea and the decrease in total number of subbasal nerve fibers in herpetic keratitis and post-refractive surgery. Tortuosity and density of cornea nerve fibers also significantly correlated with neuropathic cornea. An increase in hyperreflective keratocytes and decrease in epithelial and endothelial cells in NK eyes were observed in IVCM by Lambiase et al. (2013) [50]. However, concurrent stromal scaring, edema, infiltrate, or melting can affect the analysis of subbasal and stromal nerves plexus. Furthermore, although IVCM images can be obtained from children [51, 52], case selection and expertise in imaging are important to successfully do so.

Anterior Segment Optical Coherence Tomography (AS-OCT)

A non-contact imaging method is AS-OCT, which can be performed in children in the office or in some centers under anesthesia. The AS-OCT provides cross-sectional images of the cornea, allowing evaluation of cornea thickness at the time of NK diagnosis, as well as the monitoring of changes during disease progression or after treatment [53].

Staging and Prognosis

The severity of NK has been categorized by the Mackie classification. In stage 1, NK is characterized by cornea epitheliopathy presented as superficial punctate keratopathy. Stage 2 of NK is a progression to persistent epithelial defects and cornea erosion with the edge of persistent epithelial defect (PED) rolling. When NK advanced to stage 3, there is an ulceration with stromal lysis that can lead to cornea perforation [54]. The original Mackie classification has some limitations, for example, it does not address any changes in corneal sensitivity or stromal reactions [2, 3, 54].

Using both IVCM and AS-OCT, Mastropasua and colleagues modified the Mackie classification by taking into account the severity of subbasal nerve fibers damage as well as cellular and structural alteration in the affected cornea, with suggested prognostic and management of NK (Table 8.4) [55].

The American Society of Cataract and Refractive Surgery (ASCRS) neurotrophic keratopathy study group recently proposed an expanded staging of NK (Table 8.5) [56]. With the aim to encourage earlier detection of NK and prevent disease progression, this new and expanded staging system allows a more refined description of earlier stages of disease when corneal changes are less severe and likely more reversible. While the stage system has yet to be validated, it may be a useful tool among pediatric patients since early diagnosis and prompt treatment of NK before stromal haze would be less likely to cause any significant stromal scarring, and therefore theoretically may allow reversal of clinical signs before amblyopia develops.

Table 8.4 IVCM and OCT findings in associated with Mackie classification. Adapted from Mastropasqua et al. (2019) [55]

Classification of NK	IVCM	AS-OCT
Stage 1 (mild): • Rose Bengal or lissamine green staining of the inferior palpebral conjunctiva • Decrease tear break-up time • Increase mucous viscosity • Punctate cornea epithelial fluorescein staining	• Diffuse irregularity with increase cellular reflectivity, loss of normal epithelial stratification, focal interruption of superficial and basal layer • Increased reflectivity of the extracellular matrix • Posterior stroma appears normal in terms of transparency of the extracellular matrix (ECM) and keratocytes density	• Diffuse irregularity of epithelial surface and increased reflectivity of the epithelium and anterior stroma • No alteration or interruptions of Bowman's membrane • Stromal thickness was preserved without a sign of corneal thinning
Stage 2 (moderate) • Epithelial defect—Oval and in the central/superior cornea • Defect surrounded by a rim of loose epithelium • Edge may become smooth and rolled • Stromal swelling with folds in the Descemet's membrane • Sometime anterior chamber inflammatory reaction can be presented	• Absence of all epithelial layer with an exposition of the anterior cornea stroma • Nerve fibers were not detectable in the layer underlying epithelial defect • Anterior stroma: Presence of activated keratocytes, honeycomb-shaped edema with increased reflectivity of the ECM • Posterior stroma: Keratocyte density, transparency of ECM, tissue reflectivity, and endothelial cell count are normal • In area surrounding the lesion, epithelium is normally stratified. Anterior and posterior stroma showed normal transparency of ECM, and normal values of keratocyte density	• On area of lesion, there is interruption of the epithelial layer with typical features of crimped margins without thinning of the cornea stroma without signs of cornea ulceration • Increased reflectivity of the anterior stroma
Stage 3 (severe) • Stromal lysis or melting • Cornea perforation	• In pathological area, absence of cornea epithelial cells, basal lamina, and Bowman's membrane • An increase reflectivity of stromal tissues suggesting the presence the diffuse collagen melting, edema and tissue necrosis • Significant reduction of nerve fibers density or no nerves were detectable • Significant reduction in keratocyte density or not detectable in the lesion area • In the surrounding area of lesion, epithelium irregularity with alteration of physiological stratification, hyper-reflectivity, and desquamation of superficial cells, focal interruption of basal layer cells, and discontinuity of basal lamina	• Presence of stromal thinning in variable degree

Table 8.5 ASCRS neurotrophic keratitis study group proposed staging scheme. Adapted from Mah et al. (2021) [56]

Stage	Clinical features
0	Alteration sensation without any keratopathy
1	Cornea epitheliopathy without any stromal involvement
2	Cornea epitheliopathy with anterior stromal haze
3	Persistent or recurrent epithelial defects
4	Persistent or recurrent epithelial defects with stromal scarring, but no ulceration
5	Persistent or recurrent epithelial defects with corneal ulceration
6	Corneal perforation

Therapeutic Options and Challenges

Similar to adult disease, treatment of NK in the pediatric population is based on the clinical staging. Early diagnosis and aggressive treatment are key in the prevention of complications such as corneal scarring, the latter of which could result in permanent reduction of visual acuity from the corneal opacity as well as amblyopia in young children in whom visual development is ongoing [31].

For all stages of NK, the basic standard of care according to the expert consensus including the cessation of all preservative containing eyedrops. For eyedrops that are not available in a preservative free form, the frequency of usage should be decreased to the minimum. In addition, topical preservative free artificial tears (drop, gels, or ointments) and punctal occlusion should be considered to preserve the tear film and prevent ocular surface desiccation [3].

Medical Treatment

Traditionally, treatment of NK depends on the Mackie staging. In stage 1, treatment is aimed at preserving the epithelial integrity and preventing epithelial breakdown; in stages 2 and 3, the aim is to promote epithelial healing and prevent corneal stromal melting and perforation [54].

Preserving epithelial integrity: In mild cases of NK, the focus of treatment is to maintain epithelial stability and improve ocular surface. This is achieved by aggressive lubrication with preservative free medications either tear drops, gels, or ointment. Punctal occlusion either with plugs or via cauterization could also be considered, and these techniques have been proven safe and effective in children. Meanwhile, cessation of all offending eyedrops, such as preservative containing medications, nonsteroidal anti-inflammatory agents, and topical anesthetics should be considered [3]. In the presence of ocular surface inflammation, corticosteroids can be added. Novel therapies such as serum eyedrops may also be considered (see next section).

Epithelial defect: Once an epithelial defect has developed, additional treatment to promote ocular surface healing should be added to protect the weak or loose healing epithelium. This could be done with a therapeutic contact lens that will safeguard the epithelium from blink trauma and other environmental factors. In some children, a scleral contact lens could instead be used to provident longer-term protection of the ocular surface. In addition, topical preservative free antibiotics (e.g., moxifloxacin) is added to prevent secondary infection.

Preventing stromal lysis: In case of a neurotrophic ulcer with stromal melting, additional interventions should be urgently considered. In adult patients, systemic tetracyclines are used for their anti-inflammatory properties and their ability in the inhibition and prevention of the expression of metalloproteinase. It is important to note that in the pediatric population, especially in those under the age of 8, systemic tetracyclines can cause staining of the teeth when given more than 3 g a day for more than 10 days [31].

Novel Medical Therapies

Serum eyedrops: Autologous serum eye drops have similar osmolarity, pH, and composition to natural tears. Furthermore, they contain many ingredients like vitamins and growth factors (e.g., nerve growth factor, insulin-like growth factor, and substance-P) that have been proven helpful in the treatment of NK by promoting wound healing and optimizing the ocular surface environment for cell growth [40].

However, obtaining autologous serum eyedrops from children is undoubtedly challenging. As such, serum drops derived from allogeneic sources such as peripheral blood from parents and umbilical cord blood could be considered. Allogenic serum tears are comparable to autologous serum drops in that both have lubricant properties and contain many important tear components that promote the ocular surface to heal, including epidermal growth factor, transforming growth factor, vitamin A, and IGF-1. Both forms of allogeneic serum eyedrops are rich in growth factors [40, 57]. In the case series reported by Kalhorn et al., maternal allogenic serum drops help children with ocular surface disease resistant to multiple other treatments to heal without reporting any adverse effects [57].

Amniotic membrane: Amniotic membrane has been widely used for the treatment of ocular surface disease since 1990. The usefulness of amniotic membrane has been attributed to its anti-inflammatory, anti-scarring, anti-vascularization, anti-fibrotic effect. It is often secured with sutures or with fibrin adhesive [58]. Prokera (Bio-Tissue Inc. Doral, FL) is a suture-less cryopreserved amniotic membrane clipped to a ring system. It acts as a biological bandage. The Prokera device obviates the need for sutures and operating room, and this could be advantageous in older children who can tolerate the insertion with topical anesthesia.

Emerging Medications: Nerve Growth Factor (NGF)

Multiple in vitro studies have demonstrated that NGF is effective in signaling corneal epithelial cells for differentiation and proliferation as well as playing a role in maintaining healthy limbal stem cells. In vivo studies have showed that NGF plays a role in promoting corneal healing and induce an increase in corneal sensitivity.

Tan et al. (2006) first reported the successful treatment of NK in the pediatric population with the use of a murine nerve growth factor in a 5-month-old with bilateral neurotrophic ulcer caused by secondary congenital trigeminal insufficiency [59].

Cenegermin (Oxervate, Dompè) is a recombinant human NGF derived from *E.coli*, and it has been at the center of attention for the treatment of NK. The safety and efficacy of cenegermin were assessed in the REPARO trial, a phase I/II randomized, double masked, multicenter, parallel group study. In the phase I study, 18 adult patients with stage II or III NK were treated with recombinant NGF, and it was found that the medication was well tolerated with minor adverse effects of ocular discomfort [31, 60, 61]. In the phase II study that followed, 156 adult patients were randomized to receive either 10 µg/mL cenegermin, 20 µg/mL cenegermin, or a vehicle lubricating eyedrop. The most common cause of NK in this study was herpetic keratopathy (44/156) followed by dry eye disease (17/156). Compared to the control group, those receiving cenegermin are significantly more likely to achieve corneal epithelial healing. Only mild adverse effects were reported and there was a positive benefit to risk ratio for patients with stage 2 and 3 NK [60, 61]. After similar results were reported in the United States pivotal trial (NGF0212 and NGF0214), cenegermin was approved by the US FDA for the treatment of NK for patient over 2 years of age.

Since the FDA approval of cenegermin, there has been a number of reports in the literature describing successful treatment with of NK in the pediatric population. Pedrotti et al. reported in a one-year-old child with NK and persistent epithelial defect following surgical resection of rhabdomyosarcoma in the jaw [62]. An important report is the retrospective case series by Hatcher and colleagues (2021) in which 8 pediatric NK patients were treated with cenegermin [63]. Among them, 63% of patients (5/8) completed the entire treatment course and they all had a clinical improvement. Most recently, objective demonstration of corneal reinnervation in a case of pediatric NK was shown by Niruthisard & Fung [64]. While the questions on the long-term effects of cenegermin remain, a question particularly important for the pediatric cohort, these findings provide at least some support for the treatment of the pediatric population with cenegermin.

Surgical Treatment

Tarsorrhaphy: With more advanced disease that involves the corneal stroma (Mackie stages 2 and 3), surgical treatment may be required. Traditionally, surgical options for NK include tarsorrhaphy and conjunctival flap. In the pediatric population especially in children within the amblyogenic age range, while a permanent central or complete tarsorrhaphy and conjunctival flaps should be avoided, a temporary central tarsorrhaphy could be useful in whom an epithelial defect recalcitrant to medical treatment is present [31].

However, the authors strongly advocate the placement of a permanent *lateral* tarsorrhaphy that does not occlude the visual axis in the treatment of NK in children. A lateral tarsorrhaphy has long been proven to be effective in the management of NK [65]. In view of the lack of long-term evidence of efficacy in many of the treatment modalities, the placement of a lateral tarsorrhaphy in a single session of general anesthesia is often the most effective method in preventing disease progression, avoiding sight-threatening complications, and reducing the need for repeated examination under anesthesia in case of treatment failure thereafter.

Amniotic membrane: Another effective treatment is amniotic membrane transplant, either single or multilayer sutured to the ocular surface. This has been showed to be effective in helping epithelial healing in greater than 70% of patients. The rationale of the use of amniotic membrane has been discussed above [31, 66]. Apart from promoting epithelial healing, multilayer amniotic membrane transplant can also help to enhance tectonic support in cases of stromal melting.

Corneal transplant: In case of complications of NK that result in corneal scarring and visual loss, or stromal melting that threatens the integrity of the globe, corneal transplant either as full thickness penetrating keratoplasty or partial thickness anterior lamellar Keratoplasty could be considered. While a detailed review of pediatric keratoplasty is beyond the scope of this review, several precautions must be considered. Firstly, corneal transplant in the setting of adult NK has a high risk of complications (such as non-healing epithelial defect) and graft failure, and this is no different in children. A combination of keratoplasty, amniotic membrane overlay, and permanent lateral tarsorrhaphy, with a possible supplementary temporary central tarsorrhaphy may help to reduce the occurrence of early postoperative complications. Second, corneal transplant in children is known to carry a higher risk of graft rejection and failure long after the primary surgery, and intensive and careful monitoring is key. Finally, amblyopia treatment is paramount to ensure good visual outcome after keratoplasty.

Novel Intervention: Corneal Neurotization

Corneal neurotization refers to sensory reinnervation in neurotrophic keratopathy, first described in 2009 by Terzis et al. [67]. The procedure since its first description has been modified and can be categorized as two different approaches, the direct and indirect approach. The direct approach constitutes re-routing sensory nerves to the diseased cornea; the indirect route uses either allogenic or autologous nerves to connect the cornea with an intact sensory nerve [31, 68].

Direct neurotization: In the original description of this technique published by Terzis et al. [67], the procedure involves a bicoronal incision that transect from one ear and advances superior to the other side. The layers of scalp are then reflected to allow identification and isolation of the contralateral supratrochlear and supraorbital nerves. Once dissected, these nerves are tunneled across the nasal bridge and externalized through an eyelid crease incision over the ipsilateral affected cornea. In the six eyes which underwent this procedure, all showed improvement in visual acuity, sensibility, and progression of neurotrophic keratopathy.

However, direct neurotization has several limitations. The procedure requires an extensive dissection, with associated large area of denervation over the scalp and alopecia. As such, the technique initially failed to gain traction until it was revisited recently. A less invasive endoscopic approach have since been developed to perform the nerve dissection within the subperiosteal and subgaleal planes [69]. Another variation is to utilize the ipsilateral infraorbital nerve as a donor, which although negates the issue of scalp dissection is associated with a large area of sensory denervation over the maxillary area involving the lower eyelid, the side of the nostril, and the upper lip. All the direct neurotization techniques are also suitable for unilateral disease only. This is an important consideration in pediatric NK, as bilateral conditions are more frequently encountered.

Indirect neurotization: First developed by Ali, Borchel and Zuker in 2014, this technique uses interpositional nerve autografts to connect donor nerve to the affected neurotrophic cornea [70]. Termed minimally invasive corneal neurotization, this technique negates the need for any scalp incisions or large scalp denervation. It also allows for the treatment of bilateral neurotrophic keratopathy. The preferred donor nerve harvested is the sural nerve, but the great auricular nerve and the lateral antebrachial cutaneous nerve have also been used [69].

Since its publication, there have been multiple case reports and case series in literature involving both adult and pediatric patients, using different nerve grafts and donor nerve roots (see Table 8.6).

One of largest pediatric cohorts remains the one by the Toronto group [52, 72]. In the earlier report in which 16 patients were followed over a 5-year period [52], 15 (88%) of the patients were less than 18 years old. Following indirect corneal neurotization, central corneal sensation significantly improved at both 6 months and at final follow-up.

In the latest follow-up report by Woo et al., the pediatric cohort was expanded to 17 patients along with 6 adult patients. Overall, 14 patients (60.9%) had congenital corneal anesthesia. Mean BCVA significantly improved by 12 months after surgery. The authors also found that patients who achieved higher central corneal sensation $\geq$50 mm are less likely to develop corneal epithelial defects in the postoperative period. Furthermore, they determined that those with a shorter denervation time (<60 months) and those with $\leq$3 fascicle inserted intraoperatively are more likely to result in higher central corneal sensation. In support, Park et al. investigated the

Table 8.6 Summary of studies of cornea neurotization in pediatric population. Adapted from Solyman et al. (2022) [71]

Citation	Number of patients	Age at diagnosis of denervation	Age at neurotization surgery	Technique	Improved sensation	Time to sensation recovery
Elbaz et al. [70] Catapano et al. [52] Woo et al. [72]	28 eyes of 23 patients (22 eyes of 18 children)	77.4 ± 60.8 months	9 years	Sural nerve graft connecting to supratrochlear ad supraorbital nerve (end-to-end and contralateral)	Yes	11.1 ± 6.2 months Median 9 months
Sepehripour et al. [73]	1 of 1 child	0/months	2 years	Sural nerve graft connecting to contralateral supratrochlear nerve	Yes	2 months
Leyngold et al. [74]	1 eye of 1 child (out of 7 patients)	0/months	6 years	Acellular nerve allograft connecting to contralateral supraorbital nerve	Yes	6 months
Ebner et al. [75]	1 child	11 years	14 years	Sural nerve graft end-to-end to contralateral supraorbital nerve	Yes	4 months
Lathrop et al. [76]	1 child	8 years	13 years	Sural nerve graft end-to-end to contralateral supratrochlear nerve	Yes	3 months

outcomes of indirect corneal neurotization by age and found that children (0–17 years) achieved better corneal sensory ad visual outcomes compared to the adult cohorts [77]. These results suggest that children may be more likely to benefit from indirect corneal neurotization, and pediatric ophthalmologists looking after children with NK should consider referring for this procedure early in the disease course to prevent irreversible visual loss.

Sweeney et al. recently reported a case series in which 17 patients underwent cornea neurotization using processed nerve allografts [78]. In the cohort, 3 patients were children, with 2 suffering from combined trigeminal and facial nerve palsy and the remainder suffering from non-viral corneal infection. After corneal neurotization, corneal sensation improved in the child with corneal infection quantitatively, and qualitatively in one of the two children with nerve palsies. The mean time for improvement corneal sensation was approximately 5 months. The technique of using processed nerve allografts is controversial. Although the authors claimed that it is safe and highly effective, the accompanying editorial highlighted a number of scientific and regulatory issues [79]. Further studies are therefore needed in order to assess the safety and efficacy of this technique as a treatment for neurotrophic keratopathy in the pediatric population.

Direct and indirect corneal neurotization have different advantages and limitations, and although both have been shown clinically efficacious in the treatment of NK and in restoring corneal sensation, it has not been reported if one technique is superior to the other [68, 80]. Although not in the pediatric population, it is important to mention the prospective comparative study by Fogagnolo et al., in which 16 eyes undergoing direct corneal neurotization were compared with 10 eyes undergoing indirect corneal neurotization [80]. All patients had healed from NK in a mean period of 3.9 months without difference between direct and indirect surgical techniques, similar comparative studies in pediatric population are needed to assess if there is truly a superior technique in this age range.

Conclusions

Although uncommon, pediatric NK can have severe consequences if not diagnosed and treated in a timely fashion. When NK is suspected in children, both congenital and acquired causes should be considered. The key to successful management of pediatric NK is careful management of the corneal epithelial surface, either with medical treatment including aggressive preservative free lubrication and ointments, anti-inflammatory and anti-collagenolytic agents, and therapeutic contact lenses. Additionally, biological agents such as serum eyedrops and nerve growth factor have been shown to be safe and effective in pediatric NK. In contrast to adult condition, surgical treatment such as lateral tarsorrhaphy, amniotic membrane transplantation, and corneal neurotization should be considered early, so that permanent vision loss due to either stromal scarring and/or amblyopia could be minimized if not prevented.

References

1. Chang BH, Ewald MD, Groos EB Jr. Neurotrophic keratitis. In: Mannis MJ, Holland EJ, editors. Cornea: fundamentals, diagnosis and management. Elsevier: Canada; 2022. p. 946–553.
2. Dua HS, Said DG, Messmer EM, et al. Neurotrophic keratopathy. Prog Retin Eye Res. 2018;66:107–31. https://doi.org/10.1016/j.preteyeres.2018.04.003.
3. Dana R, Farid M, Gupta PK, et al. Expert consensus on the identification, diagnosis, and treatment of neurotrophic keratopathy. BMC Ophthalmol. 2021;21(1):327. https://doi.org/10.1186/s12886-021-02092-1.
4. Sacchetti M, Lambiase A. Diagnosis and management of neurotrophic keratitis. Clin Ophthalmol. 2014;8:571–9. https://doi.org/10.2147/OPTH.S45921.
5. Labetoulle M, Auquier P, Conrad H, et al. Incidence of herpes simplex virus keratitis in France. Ophthalmology. 2005;112(5):888–95. https://doi.org/10.1016/j.ophtha.2004.11.052.
6. Dworkin RH, Johnson RW, Breuer J, et al. Recommendations for the management of herpes zoster. Clin Infect Dis. 2007;44(Suppl 1):S1–S26. https://doi.org/10.1086/510206.
7. Bhatti MT, Patel R. Neuro-ophthalmic considerations in trigeminal neuralgia and its surgical treatment. Curr Opin Ophthalmol. 2005;16(6):334–40. https://doi.org/10.1097/01.icu.0000183859.67294.c6.
8. Roth M, Dierse S, Alder J, Holtmann C, Geerling G. Incidence, prevalence, and outcome of moderate to severe neurotrophic keratopathy in a German tertiary referral center from 2013 to 2017. Graefes Arch Clin Exp Ophthalmol. 2022;260(6):1961–73. https://doi.org/10.1007/s00417-021-05535-z.
9. Saad S, Abdelmassih Y, Saad R, et al. Neurotrophic keratitis: frequency, etiologies, clinical management and outcomes. Ocul Surf. 2020;18(2):231–6. https://doi.org/10.1016/j.jtos.2019.11.008.
10. Bonini S, Rama P, Olzi D, Lambiase A. Neurotrophic keratitis. Eye (Lond). 2003;17(8):989–95. https://doi.org/10.1038/sj.eye.6700616.
11. Bonini S, Lambiase A, Rama P, Caprioglio G, Aloe L. Topical treatment with nerve growth factor for neurotrophic keratitis. Ophthalmology. 2000;107(7):1347–52. https://doi.org/10.1016/s0161-6420(00)00163-9.
12. Müller LJ, Marfurt CF, Kruse F, Tervo TM. Corneal nerves: structure, contents and function. [published correction appears in Exp eye res. 2003 Aug;77(2):253]. Exp Eye Res. 2003;76(5):521–42. https://doi.org/10.1016/s0014-4835(03)00050-2.
13. Zander E, Weddell G. Observations on the innervation of the cornea. J Anat. 1951;85(1):68–99.
14. Yang AY, Chow J, Liu J. Corneal innervation and sensation: the eye and beyond. Yale J Biol Med. 2018;91(1):13–21. Published 2018 Mar 28
15. Marfurt CF, Kingsley RE, Echtenkamp SE. Sensory and sympathetic innervation of the mammalian cornea. A retrograde tracing study. Invest Ophthalmol Vis Sci. 1989;30(3):461–72.
16. Shaheen BS, Bakir M, Jain S. Corneal nerves in health and disease. Surv Ophthalmol. 2014;59(3):263–85. https://doi.org/10.1016/j.survophthal.2013.09.002.
17. Acosta MC, Peral A, Luna C, Pintor J, Belmonte C, Gallar J. Tear secretion induced by selective stimulation of corneal and conjunctival sensory nerve fibers. Invest Ophthalmol Vis Sci. 2004;45(7):2333–6. https://doi.org/10.1167/iovs.03-1366.
18. Versura P, Giannaccare G, Pellegrini M, Sebastiani S, Campos EC. Neurotrophic keratitis: current challenges and future prospects. Eye Brain. 2018;10:37–45. Published 2018 Jun 28. https://doi.org/10.2147/EB.S117261.
19. Sacchetti M, Micera A, Lambiase A, et al. Tear levels of neuropeptides increase after specific allergen challenge in allergic conjunctivitis. Mol Vis. 2011;17:47–52. Published 2011 Jan 7
20. Mastropasqua L, Massaro-Giordano G, Nubile M, Sacchetti M. Understanding the pathogenesis of neurotrophic keratitis: the role of corneal nerves. J Cell Physiol. 2017;232(4):717–24. https://doi.org/10.1002/jcp.25623.
21. Ramaesh K, Stokes J, Henry E, Dutton GN, Dhillon B. Congenital corneal anesthesia. Surv Ophthalmol. 2007;52(1):50–60. https://doi.org/10.1016/j.survophthal.2006.10.004.

22. Mantelli F, Nardella C, Tiberi E, Sacchetti M, Bruscolini A, Lambiase A. Congenital corneal anesthesia and neurotrophic keratitis: diagnosis and management. Biomed Res Int. 2015;2015:1. https://doi.org/10.1155/2015/805876.

23. Rosenberg ML. Congenital trigeminal anaesthesia. A review and classification. Brain. 1984;107(Pt 4):1073–82. https://doi.org/10.1093/brain/107.4.1073.

24. Gelzinis A, Simonaviciute D, Krucaite A, Buzzonetti L, Dollfus H, Zemaitiene R. Neurotrophic keratitis due to congenital corneal anesthesia with deafness, hypotonia, intellectual disability, face abnormality and metabolic disorder: a new syndrome? Medicina (Kaunas). 2022;58(5):657. https://doi.org/10.3390/medicina58050657.

25. Kamal SM, Riccobono K, Kwok A, Edmond JC, Pflugfelder SC. Unilateral pediatric neurotrophic keratitis due to congenital left trigeminal nerve aplasia with PROSE (prosthetic replacement of the ocular surface ecosystem) treatment. Am J Ophthalmol Case Rep. 2020;20:100854. Published 2020 Aug 3. https://doi.org/10.1016/j.ajoc.2020.100854.

26. Morishige N, Morita Y, Yamada N, Nishida T, Sonoda KH. Congenital hypoplastic trigeminal nerve revealed by manifestation of corneal disorders likely caused by neural factor deficiency. Case Rep Ophthalmol. 2014;5(2):181–5. https://doi.org/10.1159/000364899.

27. Rollon-Mayordomo A, Mataix-Albert B, Espejo-Arjona F, et al. Neurotrophic keratitis in a pediatric patient with Goldenhar syndrome and trigeminal aplasia successfully treated by corneal Neurotization. Ophthalmic Plast Reconstr Surg. 2022;38(2):e49–51. https://doi.org/10.1097/IOP.0000000000002086.

28. Sethi A, Ramasubramanian S, Swaminathan M. The painless eye: neurotrophic keratitis in a child suffering from hereditary sensory autonomic neuropathy type IV. Indian J Ophthalmol. 2020;68(10):2270–2. https://doi.org/10.4103/ijo.IJO_2101_19.

29. Soifer M, Gomez-Caraballo M, Venkateswaran N, Jay GW, Perez VL. Associated neurotrophic keratopathy in complex regional pain syndrome. Cornea. 2021;40(12):1600–3. https://doi.org/10.1097/ICO.0000000000002684.

30. Lambley RG, Pereyra-Muñoz N, Parulekar M, Mireskandari K, Ali A. Structural and functional outcomes of anaesthetic cornea in children. Br J Ophthalmol. 2015;99(3):418–24. https://doi.org/10.1136/bjophthalmol-2014-305719.

31. Scelfo C, Mantagos IS. Neurotrophic keratopathy in pediatric patients. Semin Ophthalmol. 2021;36(4):289–95. https://doi.org/10.1080/08820538.2021.1896747.

32. Serna-Ojeda JC, Ramirez-Miranda A, Navas A, Jimenez-Corona A, Graue-Hernandez EO. Herpes Simplex Virus Disease of the Anterior Segment in Children. [published correction appears in Cornea. 2015 Nov;34(11):e37]. Cornea. 2015;34(Suppl 10):S68–71. https://doi.org/10.1097/ICO.0000000000000559.

33. Vadoothker S, Andrews L, Jeng BH, Levin MR. Management of Herpes Simplex Virus Keratitis in the pediatric population. Pediatr Infect Dis J. 2018;37(9):949–51. https://doi.org/10.1097/INF.0000000000002114.

34. Weinmann S, Chun C, Schmid DS, et al. Incidence and clinical characteristics of herpes zoster among children in the varicella vaccine era, 2005–2009. J Infect Dis. 2013;208(11):1859–68. https://doi.org/10.1093/infdis/jit405.

35. Krall P, Kubal A. Herpes zoster stromal keratitis after varicella vaccine booster in a pediatric patient. Cornea. 2014;33(9):988–9. https://doi.org/10.1097/ICO.0000000000000199.

36. Kunimoto DY, Sharma S, Reddy MK, et al. Microbial keratitis in children. Ophthalmology. 1998;105(2):252–7. https://doi.org/10.1016/s0161-6420(98)92899-8.

37. Rubino P, Mora P, Ungaro N, Gandolfi SA, Orsoni JG. Anterior segment findings in vitamin a deficiency: a case series. Case Rep Ophthalmol Med. 2015;2015:181267. https://doi.org/10.1155/2015/181267.

38. Nassiri N, Assarzadegan F, Shahriari M, et al. Vitamin B12 deficiency as a cause of neurotrophic keratopathy. Open Ophthalmol J. 2018;12:7–11. Published 2018 Feb 28. https://doi.org/10.2174/1874364101712010007.

39. Trope GE, Jay JL, Dudgeon J, Woodruff G. Self-inflicted corneal injuries in children with congenital corneal anaesthesia. Br J Ophthalmol. 1985;69(7):551–4. https://doi.org/10.1136/bjo.69.7.551.

40. NaPier E, Camacho M, McDevitt TF, Sweeney AR. Neurotrophic keratopathy: current challenges and future prospects. Ann Med. 2022;54(1):666–73. https://doi.org/10.1080/0785389 0.2022.2045035.

41. Lawrenson JG, Birhah R, Murphy PJ. Tear-film lipid layer morphology and corneal sensation in the development of blinking in neonates and infants. J Anat. 2005;206(3):265–70. https://doi.org/10.1111/j.1469-7580.2005.00386.

42. Norn MS. Measurement of sensitivity. In: Norn MS, editor. External eye disease. Methods of examination. Copenhagen: Munksgaard International Publisher Ltd; 1974.

43. Golebiowski B, Papas E, Stapleton F. Assessing the sensory function of the ocular surface: implications of use of a non-contact air jet aesthesiometer versus the Cochet-bonnet aesthesiometer. Exp Eye Res. 2011;92(5):408–13. https://doi.org/10.1016/j.exer.2011.02.016.

44. Belmonte C, Gallar J. Cold thermoreceptors, unexpected players in tear production and ocular dryness sensations. Invest Ophthalmol Vis Sci. 2011;52(6):3888–92. Published 2011 Jun 1. https://doi.org/10.1167/iovs.09-5119.

45. Mandahl A. Hypertonic saline test for ophthalmic nerve impairment. Acta Ophthalmol. 1993;71(4):556–9. https://doi.org/10.1111/j.1755-3768.1993.tb04636.x.

46. Lum E, Corbett MC, Murphy PJ. Corneal sensitivity after ocular surgery. Eye Contact Lens. 2019;45(4):226–37. https://doi.org/10.1097/ICL.0000000000000543.

47. Cruzat A, Qazi Y, Hamrah P. In vivo confocal microscopy of corneal nerves in health and disease. Ocul Surf. 2017;15(1):15–47. https://doi.org/10.1016/j.jtos.2016.09.004.

48. Petroll WM, Robertson DM. In vivo confocal microscopy of the cornea: new developments in image acquisition, reconstruction, and analysis using the HRT-Rostock corneal module. Ocul Surf. 2015;13(3):187–203. https://doi.org/10.1016/j.jtos.2015.05.002.

49. Dhillon VK, Elalfy MS, Al-Aqaba M, Gupta A, Basu S, Dua HS. Corneal hypoesthesia with normal sub-basal nerve density following surgery for trigeminal neuralgia. Acta Ophthalmol. 2016;94(1):e6–e10. https://doi.org/10.1111/aos.12697.

50. Lambiase A, Sacchetti M, Mastropasqua A, Bonini S. Corneal changes in neurosurgically induced neurotrophic keratitis. JAMA Ophthalmol. 2013;131(12):1547–53. https://doi.org/10.1001/jamaophthalmol.2013.5064.

51. Fung SSM, Catapano J, Elbaz U, Zuker RM, Borschel GH, Ali A. In vivo confocal microscopy reveals corneal Reinnervation after treatment of neurotrophic keratopathy with corneal Neurotization. Cornea. 2018;37(1):109–12. https://doi.org/10.1097/ICO.0000000000001315.

52. Catapano J, Fung SSM, Halliday W, et al. Treatment of neurotrophic keratopathy with minimally invasive corneal neurotisation: long-term clinical outcomes and evidence of corneal reinnervation. Br J Ophthalmol. 2019;103(12):1724–31. https://doi.org/10.1136/bjophthalmol-2018-313042.

53. Nubile M, Dua HS, Lanzini M, et al. In vivo analysis of stromal integration of multilayer amniotic membrane transplantation in corneal ulcers. Am J Ophthalmol. 2011;151(5):809–822.e1. https://doi.org/10.1016/j.ajo.2010.11.002.

54. Mackie IA. Neuroparalytic keratitis. In: Fraunfelder F, Roy FH, Meyer SM, editors. Current ocular therapy. Philadelphia: WB Saunders; 1995.

55. Mastropasqua L, Nubile M, Lanzini M, Calienno R, Dua HS. In vivo microscopic and optical coherence tomography classification of neurotrophic keratopathy. J Cell Physiol. 2019;234(5):6108–15. https://doi.org/10.1002/jcp.27345.

56. Mah FS, Farid M, Khandelwal S, Yeu E. Neurotrophic keratitis: a "rare disease" yet common problem. Supplement to cataract & refractive surgery today. Radnor: Evolve Medical Education; 2021.

57. Kalhorn AJ, Tawse KL, Shah AA, Jung JL, Gregory DG, McCourt EA. Maternal serum eye drops in the Management of Pediatric Persistent Corneal Epithelial Defects: a case series. Cornea. 2018;37(7):912–5. https://doi.org/10.1097/ICO.0000000000001512.

58. Suri K, Kosker M, Raber IM, et al. Sutureless amniotic membrane ProKera for ocular surface disorders: short-term results. Eye Contact Lens. 2013;39(5):341–7. https://doi.org/10.1097/ICL.0b013e3182a2f8fa.

59. Tan MH, Bryars J, Moore J. Use of nerve growth factor to treat congenital neurotrophic corneal ulceration. Cornea. 2006;25(3):352–5. https://doi.org/10.1097/01.ico.0000176609.42838.df.

60. Bonini S, Lambiase A, Rama P, et al. Phase I trial of recombinant human nerve growth factor for neurotrophic keratitis. Ophthalmology. 2018;125(9):1468–71. https://doi.org/10.1016/j.ophtha.2018.03.004.

61. Bonini S, Lambiase A, Rama P, et al. Phase II randomized, double-masked, vehicle-controlled trial of recombinant human nerve growth factor for neurotrophic keratitis. Ophthalmology. 2018;125(9):1332–43. https://doi.org/10.1016/j.ophtha.2018.02.022.

62. Pedrotti E, Bonetto J, Cozzini T, Fasolo A, Marchini G. Cenegermin in pediatric neurotrophic keratopathy. Cornea. 2019;38(11):1450–2. https://doi.org/10.1097/ICO.0000000000002112.

63. Hatcher JB, Soifer M, Morales NG, Farooq AV, Perez VL, Shieh C. Aftermarket effects of cenegermin for neurotrophic keratopathy in pediatric patients. Ocul Surf. 2021;21:52–7. https://doi.org/10.1016/j.jtos.2021.04.003.

64. Niruthisard D, Fung S. Recombinant human nerve growth factor for pediatric neurotrophic keratopathy. Eye Contact Lens. 2022;48:10–1097. https://doi.org/10.1097/ICL.0000000000000912.

65. Trinh T, Mimouni M, Santaella G, Cohen E, Chan CC. Surgical Management of the Ocular Surface in neurotrophic keratopathy: amniotic membrane, conjunctival grafts, lid surgery, and Neurotization. Eye Contact Lens. 2021;47(3):149–53. https://doi.org/10.1097/ICL.0000000000000753.

66. Chen HJ, Pires RT, Tseng SC. Amniotic membrane transplantation for severe neurotrophic corneal ulcers. Br J Ophthalmol. 2000;84(8):826–33. https://doi.org/10.1136/bjo.84.8.826.

67. Terzis JK, Dryer MM, Bodner BI. Corneal neurotization: a novel solution to neurotrophic keratopathy. Plast Reconstr Surg. 2009;123(1):112–20. https://doi.org/10.1097/PRS.0b013e3181904d3a.

68. Wolkow N, Habib LA, Yoon MK, Freitag SK. Corneal Neurotization: review of a new surgical approach and its developments. Semin Ophthalmol. 2019;34(7–8):473–87. https://doi.org/10.1080/08820538.2019.1648692.

69. Liu CY, Arteaga AC, Fung SE, Cortina MS, Leyngold IM, Aakalu VK. Corneal neurotization for neurotrophic keratopathy: review of surgical techniques and outcomes. Ocul Surf. 2021;20:163–72. https://doi.org/10.1016/j.jtos.2021.02.010.

70. Elbaz U, Bains R, Zuker RM, Borschel GH, Ali A. Restoration of corneal sensation with regional nerve transfers and nerve grafts: a new approach to a difficult problem. JAMA Ophthalmol. 2014;132(11):1289–95. https://doi.org/10.1001/jamaophthalmol.2014.2316.

71. Solyman O, Elhusseiny AM, Ali SF, Allen R. A review of pediatric corneal Neurotization. Int Ophthalmol Clin. 2022;62(1):83–94. https://doi.org/10.1097/IIO.0000000000000403.

72. Woo JH, Christian DS, Kamiar M, Howard BG, Asim A. Minimally invasive corneal neurotization provides sensory function, protects against recurrent ulceration, and improves visual acuity. [published online ahead of print, 2022 May 2]. Am J Ophthalmol. 2022;241:179–89. https://doi.org/10.1016/j.ajo.2022.04.013.

73. Sepehripour S, Lloyd MS, Nishikawa H, et al. Surrogates outcomes measures for corneal neurotization in infants and children. J Craniofacial surgery. 2017;28:1167–70.

74. Leyngold IM, Yen MT, Tian J, et al. Minimally corneal neurotization with acellular nerve allograft: Surgical techniques and clinical outcomes. Ophthal Plast Reconstru Surg. 2019:35:133–40.

75. Ebner R, Fridirich G, Sokolovsky M, et al. In vivo corneal confocal microscopy: pre-and post-operative evaluation in a case of corneal neurotization. Neurophthalmology. 2019:44:193–6.

76. Lathrop KL, Duncan K, Yu J, et al. Development of corneal sensation with remodeling of the epithelium and the palisades of vogt after corneal neurotization. Cornea 2020:39:657–60.

77. Park JK, Charlson ES, Leyngold I, Kossler AL. Corneal Neurotization: a review of pathophysiology and outcomes. Ophthalmic Plast Reconstr Surg. 2020;36(5):431–7. https://doi.org/10.1097/IOP.0000000000001583.

78. Sweeney AR, Wang M, Weller CL, et al. Outcomes of corneal neurotisation using processed nerve allografts: a multicentre case series. Br J Ophthalmol. 2022;106(3):326–30. https://doi.org/10.1136/bjophthalmol-2020-317361.
79. Jowett N, Pineda R 2nd. Corneal and facial sensory Neurotization in trigeminal anesthesia. Acellular nerve allografts in corneal neurotisation: an inappropriate choice. Br J Ophthalmol. 2020;104(2):149–50. https://doi.org/10.1136/bjophthalmol-2019-315032.
80. Fogagnolo P, Giannaccare G, Bolognesi F, et al. Direct versus indirect corneal Neurotization for the treatment of neurotrophic keratopathy: a multicenter prospective comparative study. Am J Ophthalmol. 2020;220:203–14. https://doi.org/10.1016/j.ajo.2020.07.003.

Chapter 9
The Role of Contact Lenses in the Management of Ocular Surface Disease in Children

Karen G. Carrasquillo (iD), Daniel Brocks (iD), Nathan Lollins Cheung (iD), and Kellen Riccobono (iD)

Introduction

Though once believed to be less common, pediatric ocular surface disease is regularly identified at the slit lamp by optometrists and ophthalmologists in modern day practice [1]. Ambient environment and daily activities such as smartphone and computer usage may be important factors [2]. Though ocular surface disease in the pediatric population most frequently refers to the general category of dry eye disease, other less common pathologies such as neurotrophic keratitis, limbal stem cell deficiency, ocular rosacea, contact lens induced ocular surface disease and exposure keratitis may be regularly seen in the clinic setting, particularly in a referral center [3–6]. Additionally, ocular surface disease in the pediatric population may frequently be under-recognized [7, 8].

The use of bandage contact lenses and scleral lenses for the management of ocular surface disease is highlighted in the TFOS DEWS II Report as a "Step 3" treatment option for dry eye disease [9]. However, and of note, neither the full TFOS nor the executive summary mentions either bandage contact lens or scleral lens use in the context of pediatric ocular surface disease management [9, 10]. Typically, most pediatric ocular surface disease care is extrapolated from clinical trials with

K. G. Carrasquillo · D. Brocks (✉)
BostonSight, Needham, MA, USA
e-mail: kcarrasquillo@bostonsight.org; dbrocks@bostonsight.org

N. L. Cheung
Department of Pediatric Ophthalmology, Duke University, Durham, NC, USA
e-mail: Nathan.cheung@duke.edu

K. Riccobono
Cornea and Contact Lens Department, New England College of Optometry, Boston, MA, USA
e-mail: kriccobono@ctectx.com

enrollment of subjects 18 years of age or older. When utilizing the TFOS DEWS II Report, it is therefore most sensible and understandable that clinicians tend to gravitate toward more conservative measures for the pediatric population that involve lower risk and fewer obstacles to implementation. Most certainly, modification of local environment when possible, and interventions such as lubricating drops or ointments and lid hygiene management are more straightforward and lower risk for a family to adopt as a treatment strategy for their young child. When these initial steps fail, it is common for the clinician to direct their attention to other medication regimens, such as topical steroids, topical lifitegrast, topical cyclosporine, topical cenegermin, or other modalities such as punctal occlusion, though many of these applications in the pediatric population are indeed off-label. For instance, the safety and efficacy of topical 0.05% cyclosporine (Restasis, Abbvie, Chicago, IL) have only been evaluated and approved by the U.S. Food and Drug Administration (FDA) for those 16 years of age or older [11]. The role of bandage contacts lenses, typically used for acute care, and the role of scleral lenses, typically used for chronic ocular surface management, in the pediatric population is often unconsidered under the assumption that too many challenges or obstacles will stand in the way of implementation, rendering this potentially highly efficacious modality underutilized.

In general, soft bandage contact lenses provide a temporary barrier to protect the ocular surface from environmental and mechanical challenges, particularly in such instances of acute corneal erosions, abrasions, or more specifically in neurotrophic disease unresponsive to lower risk options. The proper labeled use of soft bandage contact lenses and the distinction between the approved lens options currently available to the practitioner are of the utmost importance and will be reviewed in this chapter. Scleral lenses and PROSE devices (BostonSight, Needham MA) provide a long-term solution to chronic ocular surface disease, the utility and efficacy of which have been well documented for the indications of ocular surface support [12, 13]. These rigid gas permeable lenses rest solely on the conjunctiva and vault over the limbus and cornea. The preservative-free sterile normal saline filled reservoir provides a protected environment for ocular surface support while providing improved comfort and best corrected visual acuity [14]. There is often a preconceived notion that scleral lenses and PROSE devices cannot be utilized for the pediatric population. However, with the proper specialist and support, these lenses may be part of the treatment regimen for infants, children, and adolescents alike. Specific special considerations must be adopted in order to choose the appropriate patients and to successfully dispense these lenses. Most certainly, the decision to proceed with such an intervention does not come lightly and must take into account family support, patient cooperativity, specialized strategies for lens application and removal techniques and training, as well as in depth informed consent balancing carefully the risks, benefits, and alternatives.

The recent surge in the adoption of scleral lenses in the adult population will likely slowly transform into an increased utilization in pediatric eye care [15, 16]. It is notable that not only does the TFOS DEWS II Report not address the pediatric population specifically, but also there is limited literature currently available reviewing the use of bandage contact lenses or scleral lenses in pediatric optometry and ophthalmology [17–22].

This chapter will provide an overview of bandage contact lens and scleral lens indications and utilization in the management of pediatric ocular surface disease, including definitions, material options, and labeling. Special considerations when working in this arena with pediatric patients will be highlighted, including training and fitting techniques, social issues such as family involvement, contraindications, and integration with other treatment modalities. Overall, bandage contact lenses and scleral lenses can play a significant role as an option for the management of ocular surface disease in the pediatric population, however, a notable commitment can be required, not only by the patient and family, but also from a collaborative approach by the clinicians involved.

Bandage Contact Lenses

Historically the term "bandage contact lenses," also termed "therapeutic soft contact lenses," has not been well defined. A recently proposed definition describes bandage contact lenses as "lenses that are used for the treatment of ocular discomfort or to support the cornea during healing after surgery or when the cornea is being treated for an underlying disease state or to protect the cornea from the environment or mechanical interaction with the lids" [23]. Soft bandage contact lenses can serve a vital role in the management of ocular surface disease, particularly in acute settings such as corneal abrasions and corneal erosions, and after other lower risk treatment options have failed. Bandage contact lenses are cited in the DEWS II Report as a treatment approach that can be used either on a short-term or long-term basis [24]. Short-term use for acute indications is typically for a period of a few days, while long-term use for weeks, months, or even years, for chronic indications is less commonly utilized. Bandage contact lenses are typically used on an extended-wear (EW) schedule in management of acute indications, while in other cases, typically in the management of chronic indications, bandage contact lenses may be used on a daily-wear (DW) schedule [24]. The most common use of bandage contact lens is a short-term extended-wear schedule where the lens is removed after the epitheliopathy is healed, however in cases of long-term extended or daily wear, lenses should be replaced periodically at the discretion of the practitioner (such as weekly, biweekly, or monthly).

Bandage contact lenses assist in the treatment and management of ocular surface disease by providing a physical barrier to adverse environmental factors that delay healing. This includes protection from mechanical lid interaction, which can be especially important in subtypes of ocular surface disease that involve keratinization of the lid margin and/or palpebral conjunctiva such as Stevens-Johnson syndrome, lid wiper epitheliopathy, and ocular mucous membrane pemphigoid. Additionally, bandage lenses provide improved comfort for the patient during healing while also maintaining visual function, for example, in postoperative use or in the setting of a corneal abrasion.

The proposed mechanisms in which bandage contact lenses aid in corneal healing are via stabilization of the tear film and restoration of epithelial cell turnover. It is also posited that the mechanism for pain relief is by means of the insulation of sensitized corneal nerves and shielding of the nociceptors, particularly from lid and tarsal related trauma [25–27]. There is evidence to support the use of bandage contact lenses in a variety of ocular surface disease indications. For example, bandage contact lenses have led to shorter corneal ulcer healing times in non-infectious neurotrophic keratitis when compared to drops alone [28]. They are also used in moderate to severe ocular-graft-versus-host-disease with good safety, efficacy, and tolerance when other treatments have failed [28]. Indications for bandage contact lenses in pediatric patients include in cases of bullous keratopathy, corneal abrasions, epithelial erosions, or postoperatively for pain relief. Bandage contact lenses can also enhance corneal healing in cases of persistent epithelial defects, neurotrophic keratitis, chemical burns, descemetocele, and dry eye syndrome. Additionally, they can be used for corneal protection from entropion, trichiasis, tarsal scarring, or in the case of recurrent corneal erosions and can also be used for corneal sealing in perforation [28].

In regard to the use of contact lenses in the pediatric population, historically silicone contact lenses were used in pediatric aphakic patients for visual correction, but led to complications due to the hydrophobic lens surfaces and lens binding [29]. Updated and improved contact lens materials have allowed for the continued use of contact lenses in pediatric aphakic patients for visual needs and, as in the focus of this chapter, for ocular surface disease. Some contemporary practitioners may still have a preconceived notion that contact lenses should not be used in children due to concerns with hygiene, handling, and patient tolerance. However, with proper risk-benefit consideration, management, education, and follow-up, bandage contact lenses can be integral in the management of pediatric patients with ocular surface disease. This section will explore the special considerations of the use of bandage contact lenses in the pediatric population.

Contact Lens Materials

An important consideration when utilizing a bandage contact lens is material selection, especially when used in an extended-wear setting. Extended wear of bandage contact lenses is typically used because of several factors. Firstly, limiting excessive application and removal may be beneficial to reduce repeated unnecessary shearing forces on the fragile, healing corneal epithelium. Secondly, limiting the amount of handling may reduce the risk of possible contamination of the lens. Additionally, depending on the child, application and removal may be difficult and may involve parent or caregiver involvement, making daily wear impractical in some cases.

Despite its potential benefits, there are risks that are introduced with extended wear of contact lenses, including corneal edema and corneal neovascularization. To attempt to mitigate these risks, bandage contact lenses of silicone hydrogel material are the standard of care with extended wear due to their higher oxygen permeability (Dk). Lenses of the alternative material (hydrogel) fail to meet the criterion of 87.0 Fk/t (87×10^{-9} (cm $\times$ mLO2)/(s $\times$ mL $\times$ mmHg) established as the minimum oxygen permeability needed to provide the cornea with sufficient oxygen in order to avoid excessive corneal swelling during extended wear [30]. This was the criterion found to limit corneal edema to 4% overnight, which is the amount of corneal edema experienced overnight in closed-eye conditions without a contact lens. Most silicone hydrogel lenses on the market reach this criterion while hydrogel lenses do not, however, it is important to note that only a small subset of silicone hydrogel lenses are FDA approved for usage in the United States as a bandage contact lens.

Infectious or infiltrative keratitis is another potential risk with the use of bandage contact lenses, particularly when used in an extended-wear setting. In one prospective, population-based surveillance study in Australia, the annualized incidence of microbial keratitis in the setting of non-therapeutic extended wear of silicone hydrogel contact lenses was twice that of daily wear of silicone hydrogel contact lenses (25.4 per 10,000 wearers versus 11.9 per 10,000 wearers, respectively) [31]. Close monitoring for infiltrative events should be employed when utilizing any form of bandage contact lenses.

On-Label Versus Off-Label Usage

Another consideration in the use of bandage contact lenses is their approval for therapeutic use given by certain regulatory institutions, such as the FDA. Table 9.1 below summarizes the lenses on the market in the U.S. that are approved by the FDA for therapeutic use at the time of this chapter's publication. Other available lenses could be used in a therapeutic setting; however, this would be considered off-label usage and would likely need to be supported by a specific and unique indication. For example, in ophthalmology, a lens that is frequently used off-label in a

Table 9.1 FDA-approved therapeutic soft contact lenses [28, 32]

Manufacturer	Lens	Material	Replacement schedule	Dk/H20	Base curves available (mm)	Diameter (mm)
Vistakon	Acuvue Oasys	Senofilcon A	Biweekly, DW Weekly, EW	103/38	8.4 9.0	14.0
Bausch and Lomb	PureVision	Balafilcon A	Monthly, EW	91/36	8.3 8.6	14.0
Alcon	Air Optix night & day	Lotrafilcon A	Monthly, EW	140/24	8.4 8.6	13.8

DW daily wear, *EW* extended wear, *Dk* oxygen permeability, *H₂O* water content therapeutic setting is the Kontur lens (Kontur Kontact Lens, Hercules, CA). Kontur lenses offer large diameter (>15 mm) which can be helpful in settings where standard diameter lenses (13–15 mm) are not able to be retained in the eye, particularly in settings of exposure and/or poor lid function [33]. A lens that is too small in diameter or too flat may have issues with lens retention. The potential benefits of the off-label utilization of a Kontur hydrogel contact lens must be balanced with the risks of the low Dk of 18.8. This risk/benefit balance is often deemed acceptable for large diameter Kontur lens usage following keratoprosthesis surgery in order to protect the remaining epithelial tissue and promote lens retention [33].

Fitting Considerations

When fitting a bandage contact lens, an appropriate base curve to corneal curvature relationship should be maintained so that the lens does not fit too flat or too steep. There are several features that define an adequately fitting therapeutic contact lens: [33]

1. Good lens centration
2. Should not cross limbus on blinks or with changes in gaze
3. Appropriate movement with blink and/or on push-up test
4. Patient does not report lens awareness or discomfort
5. Lens retention and absence of tight lens syndrome after 1 day of wear

Additionally, it is important to ensure that there are no bubbles underneath the lens on insertion as a stagnant air bubble may cause desiccation and erosion of an already fragile epithelium in patients with ocular surface disease.

Concurrent Treatments with Bandage Contact Lenses

Adjunctive therapies that may be used with bandage contact lenses include punctal occlusion (via permanent silicone or temporary collagen punctal plugs) and non-preserved topical lubrication, antibiotics, or anti-inflammatory medications. Prophylactic topical antibiotic use is a standard recommendation due to the increased risk of infectious keratitis with extended wear. Topical moxifloxacin (Vigamox®, Alcon, Fort Worth, Texas) is typically used due to its non-preserved formulation with a dosing of four times a day. Though this combination is standard in practice, uncertainties remain regarding if topical medications can permeate through the silicone hydrogel material of the bandage contact lens. One in vitro study reported detectable levels of moxifloxacin underneath the lens 20 min after instillation; however, of note, the authors used a concentration 10-times greater than the most common commercial formulation and the diffused concentration found was less than that found in standard topical formulations [34]. Instead of dosing throughout the day, off-label, some practitioners will either pre-soak or post-soak the bandage contact lens. A pre-soaked contact lens is one that has been soaked in topical drug solution before application on eye, while a post-soaked lens is applied to the eye first followed by the practitioner applying multiple drops of the topical drug solution to the lens on eye in office [28].

Bandage Contact Lenses in Pediatric Patients: Current Literature

At the time of this chapter's publication, a review of current literature revealed only one source that specifically discusses the safety and efficacy of the therapeutic use of silicone hydrogel contact lenses in children with a variety of ocular surface or anterior segment disease [19]. In this prospective, open-ended, non-randomized study in children of the age of 2 month to 17 years old (average 9.4 years old), 29 eyes were fit into the Focus Night & Day lens (CIBA Vision, Duluth, GA) on an extended wear schedule [19]. The indications for bandage contact lens use in this study were largely ocular surface disease (corneal erosion, neurotrophic keratitis, descemetocele, corneal ulcer, exposure keratitis, vernal keratoconjunctivitis, herpetic keratitis, kerato-uveitis) or related to trauma (chemical/thermal burns, corneal perforation, perforating or non-perforating corneal wound). The average duration of contact lens wear was 17.8 days with an extensive range of 1–131 days. The authors concluded that the use of extended-wear silicone hydrogel lenses was safe and effective, with only one eye discontinuing lens wear due to increased inflammation in herpetic keratitis.

Special considerations for pediatric patients were noted in the above-mentioned study [19]. For children under the age of 4 years old, the contact lenses were fitted under sedation (5 mg diazepam via rectal tube). If the lenses were used long term, they were removed and cleaned weekly by medical staff and were replaced monthly. The follow-up schedule included daily examinations for the first 5 days and then on a weekly basis if the lenses were worn longer. The patients who wore the lenses for a longer period of time were those who had neurotrophic keratitis. This may be an indication that bandage contact lenses could be a suitable long-term treatment for children with this disease. Bandage contact lens use in this cohort was noted to provide excellent pain relief and partial pain relief in 79% and 13%, respectively, and provided complete corneal healing and partial corneal healing in 76% and 17%, respectively.

Additional published literature discusses the role of bandage contact lenses after surgery in pediatric patients. In a single-center, randomized controlled trial, silicone hydrogel bandage contact lenses after frontalis muscle flap suspension for congenital blepharoptosis were noted to be safe and effective in children aged 5–11 [35]. In this trial, the contact lenses were worn for 15 days with concurrent treatment of tobramycin 0.3% and polyvinyl alcohol drops four times a day. There are also several studies that demonstrate safety and efficacy of the use of bandage contact lens after epithelium off corneal collagen crosslinking in pediatric patients, where bandage contact lenses are typically used until the epithelial defect is healed, usually a few days, with concurrent use of topical moxifloxacin [36–38].

To speak to the above-mentioned risks with bandage contact lens use, one source from the Mayo Clinic reports the incidence of microbial keratitis in the therapeutic wear of soft contact lenses to be 13.3–20.9/10,000 per year, an increase when compared to the reported incidence of 2.2–4.1/10,000 per year for daily wear of soft contact lenses [39]. In pediatric patients specifically, the incidence of microbial keratitis is not well defined; however, in one report of 93 pediatric patients under the age of five treated for microbial keratitis in a tertiary eye center, 8.6% (8 patients) within this cohort developed microbial keratitis from contact lens use. Of these eight patients (age range: 6 months to 4 years), four were wearing bandage contact lenses due to trauma, three were in soft contact lenses for aphakia, and one was in a rigid gas permeable contact lens [40].

Contraindications

Infectious keratitis is an absolute contraindication to the use of soft bandage contact lenses. Utilization of bandage contact lenses in cases of corneal anesthesia and significant exposure keratopathy with inadequate lid movement must be carefully considered as relative contraindications [28]. Though neurotrophic keratitis patients have been successfully managed with bandage contact lenses, this patient group must have particularly close follow-up and monitoring for complications because they will be unable to self-report pain symptoms, or even be aware if the lens is dislodged or expelled from the eye, which would typically prompt a patient to return to clinic immediately [28]. It is important to note that the above list is non-exhaustive, and the risks and benefits should be analyzed on a case-by-case basis and discussed with both patient and caregiver(s) after thorough education and with proper informed consent.

Scleral Lenses

A scleral lens is defined as a lens fitted to vault over the entire cornea, including the limbus, and land on the conjunctiva overlying the sclera [41]. It is filled with sterile preservative-free saline, creating a tear lens between the ocular surface and the back surface of the lens to provide constant lubrication, visual rehabilitation, ocular surface support, as well as protection from the environment and mechanical irritation from the eyelids (Fig. 9.1).

The unique anatomy of a scleral lens provides comfort by vaulting the sensitive cornea and resting on the insensitive sclera and overlying conjunctiva. Additionally,

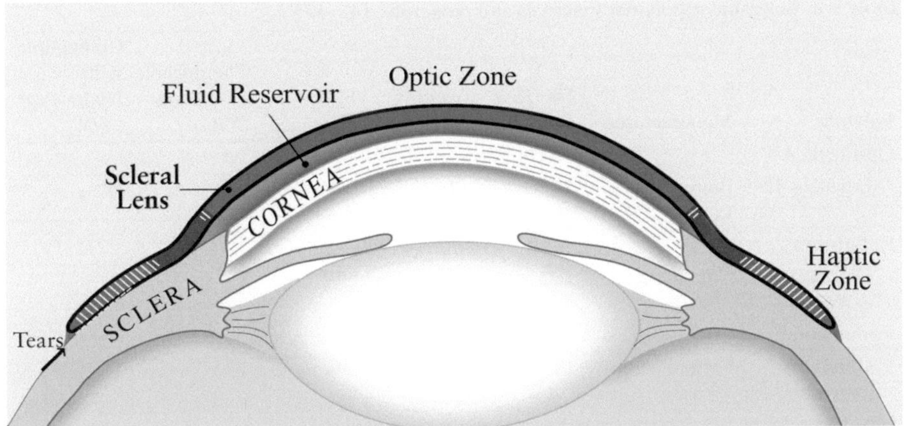

Fig. 9.1 Schematic of scleral lens on eye

the liquid reservoir that is created between the cornea and the back surface of the lens creates a microenvironment that promotes healing [42]. The rigid nature of the polymeric materials used to manufacture scleral lenses coupled with the posterior optic curve creates the fluid compartment that acts optically to nullify corneal surface irregularities, potentiating visual rehabilitation [43, 44]. Modern scleral lenses are made from fluorosilicone acrylate (FSA) polymers. The hallmark of these materials is their high Dk, although there are other notable intricate differences between the various FSA polymers, which are summarized in Table 9.2. As well, the versatile range of scleral lens diameters (14–23 mm) allows for proper customization of the pediatric population.

The three main indications for scleral lens use include:

- Visual rehabilitation
- Comfort
- Support of the ocular surface

Numerous reports describe that the positive impact scleral lenses can have across the entire spectrum of complex ocular surface disease, where there is documented improvement in visual function, activities of daily living, and quality of life [13, 52–59].

As it pertains to the pediatric patient population, scleral lenses have broad applications and benefits for both visual rehabilitation and therapeutic indications (Table 9.3) [22, 60–70]. The youngest patient reported to be fitted with scleral lenses was 7 month old [22]. Scleral lenses additionally have been shown to have a favorable safety profile, including a low incidence of microbial keratitis [71].

Scleral lenses can be especially beneficial in complex, recalcitrant cases that have failed other traditional treatment modalities or for cases with additional

Table 9.2 Scleral lens polymer materials and properties. [45–47]

Polymer	Manufacturer	Dk (ISO/ Fatt)	Wetting angle (°)	FDA clearance	Therapeutic indication (Y/N)	Compatible with Hydra-Peg[a] (Y/N)
Oprifocon A						
Equalens II[b]	Bausch & Lomb	87	30	EW[c]	Y	N
Roflufocon D						
Optimum extra	Contamac	100	<3	DW[d]	Y	Y
Roflufocon E						
Optimum extreme	Contamac	125	6	DW	Y	Y
Hexafocon A [48]						
Acuity 100	Acuity polymers	111	23	DW	N	
Boston XO	Bausch & Lomb	111	49	DW	N	Y
Hexafocon B						
Boston XO$_2$	Bausch & Lomb	141	38	DW	Y	Y
Tisilfocon A [49, 50]						
Menicon Z[e]	Menicon	163	24	CW[f]	N	N
Optimum infinite	Contamac	180	91	DW	Y	Y
Fluoroxyfocon A [51]						
Acuity 200	Acuity polymers	200	48	DW	N	Y

[a] Hydra-Peg not FDA approved for the pediatric population
[b] Approved for extended wear for orthokeratology
[c] Extended wear
[d] Daily wear
[e] First material to be approved for continuous wear (30 days). Composed of siloxanyl styrene, fluoromethacrylate, and benzotriazol, making it different than most fluorosilicone acrylate GP materials.
[f] Continuous wear

concomitant corneal disease. For instance, pediatric corneal ectasia cases are more traditionally addressed utilizing corneal gas permeable lenses, which have a higher likelihood of irritating the ocular surface. Many irregular cornea cases have concomitant ocular surface disease, such as dry eye syndrome. For these scenarios, scleral lenses may be a superior choice because of the constant lubrication rendered by the fluid reservoir and their ability to vault the cornea, both of which promote improved physiological endpoints of the ocular surface.

Table 9.3 Scleral lens indications in the pediatric population

Refractive	Irregular cornea	Ocular surface disease
Aphakia	Post trauma Keratoconus	Dry eye syndrome/Keratoconjunctivitis sicca Steven Johnsons syndrome
	Keratoglobus	Graft versus host disease

	Corneal scar	Corneal anesthesia/neurotrophic keratopathy
		    Familial dysautonomia
		    Hereditary sensory and autonomic neuropathies
		    (HSAN)
		    Secondary to herpes simplex keratitis
		    Status post radiation
		    Moebius syndrome
		    Trigeminal nerve dysfunction
		Exposure keratopathy
		    TUBB3 syndrome/congenital fibrosis of EOMs
		    Lagophthalmos
		Epidermal ocular disorders
		    Ectodermal dysplasia
		    Goldenhar syndrome

In cases of exposure keratopathy, for example, it is ideal to fit pediatric patients with as large a scleral lens as possible, considering palpebral aperture, chances for application and removal success, and the presence or absence of anatomical obstacles on the conjunctiva. This will not only protect the cornea from chronic exposure and prevent risk of further neovascularization and scarring but also will protect the conjunctival tissue from desiccation and chronic hyperemia (Fig. 9.2a). Protection from chronic desiccation and mechanical injury from lid pathology becomes especially important in cases of Stevens-Johnson Syndrome (SJS). In SJS, keratinization of the lid margins, entropion, distichiasis, and trichiasis can occur. This results in a chronic insult to the corneal and conjunctival surface. Scleral lenses not only serve as a protective barrier in these cases, but also provide much needed relief from pain and photophobia (Fig. 9.2b).

The impact of healing persistent epithelial defects in the pediatric population has been demonstrated in various scenarios in the ocular surface disease spectrum as is the case in Stevens-Johnson syndrome (Fig. 9.3a, b) and familial dysautonomia (Fig. 9.3c, d). Kamal et al. reported on the benefits that PROSE devices had in a pediatric patient with trigeminal nerve aplasia with a persistent epithelial defect that was not healed after an 8-week course of cenegermin 0.002% (Oxervate, Dompe, Milan, Italy), however, resolved with PROSE treatment with a subsequent visual acuity improvement from 20/300 to 20/70 [4]. Figure 9.3e, f shows a similar scenario, in a patient with a neurotrophic cornea, secondary to cranial nerve 6th/7th palsy after brain tumor resection, with a persistent defect that was healed with daily wear of PROSE devices.

It has been postulated that scleral lenses provide a microenvironment where healing and restoration of ocular surface functions may occur [42, 45, 72–76]. The combination of constant lubrication and protection from the environment seem to be the key elements in reducing ocular surface inflammation and promoting corneal healing

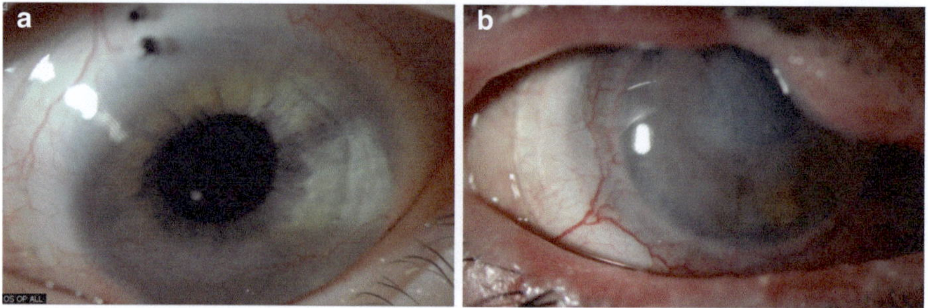

Fig. 9.2 (**a**) Large diameter scleral lens (18.0 mm) over the left eye of a pediatric patient with history of congenital fibrosis of the extraocular muscles and chronic exposure. (**b**) Scleral lens fitted over an SJS pediatric eye, protecting the cornea and ocular surface from lid margin keratinization and distichiasis. (Image courtesy of BostonSight)

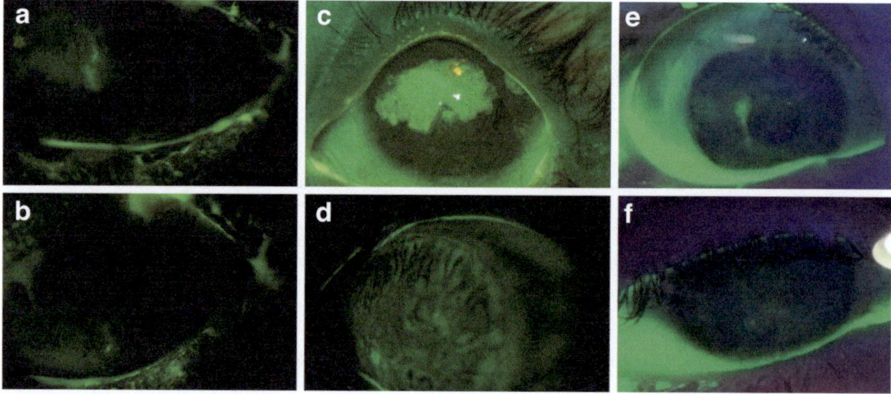

Fig. 9.3 (**a**) Epithelial defect in a pediatric patient with SJS at baseline and (**b**) after scleral lens wear. (**c**) Persistent epithelial defect in a pediatric patient with familial dysautonomia and (**d**) after scleral lens wear. (**e**) Recurrent epithelial defect after 8-week course of cenergemin in a pediatric patient with neurotrophic keratopathy from cranial nerve 6th/7th palsy after brain tumor resection and (**f**) healed after scleral lens wear. (Image courtesy of BostonSight)

and remodeling, as evidenced in some cases by the clearing of chronic corneal opacities [72–74, 76]. In their case series, Cressey et al. reported that the pediatric cases had the most dramatic improvement in corneal opacities, hypothesizing that perhaps the pediatric cornea has the greatest potential for wound healing and remodeling [72].

It is important to highlight that achieving the potential benefits of scleral lenses is dependent on adequate lens fitting mechanics. Without a proper and physiologically compatible fit, not only may these benefits not occur, but complications may ensue. As well, the choice of lens material plays a vital role in optimizing physiological endpoints, patient comfort, and satisfaction. As shown in Table 9.2, even though all materials are of high Dk, the degree of oxygen permeability varies. For severely compromised pediatric corneas and fragile endothelium, choosing the highest Dk materials available (≥140) coupled with minimizing the lens center thickness is preferred in order to reduce potential impacts of hypoxia. However, with increased oxygen permeability, there is typically an increase in hydrophobicity (due to the higher silicone content in these hyper-Dk materials), causing a decrease in lens wettability which ultimately can result in more surface lipid deposits, visually impacting wetting defects, and increased friction with blink. This trade-off calls for a fine balance to be considered when fitting a pediatric cornea with severe dry eye, such as in SJS or Graft vs Host Disease. While it is important to choose high Dk materials, in many cases opting for materials between approximately 90–100 Dk may provide the appropriate balance.

When healing recalcitrant persistent epithelial defects, some practitioners direct patients to sleep with the scleral lens for a 24 h period or provide the patient with two scleral lens which they exchange every 12 h (commonly referred to as "12/12 wear"). When utilizing any of these off-label wearing schedules, the addition of a drop of preservative-free antibiotic (such as moxifloxacin) in the fluid-reservoir as prophylaxis is a standard approach. Any treatment course of this nature most certainly requires a thorough informed consent process with the parent/legal guardian prior to initiation, which includes an extensive discussion of the risks, benefits, and alternatives [76, 77]. All pediatric patients must be monitored extremely closely in clinic when such regimens are implemented.

Special Considerations

Training: Application and Removal

Contact lenses can only be used in the pediatric population if the contact lens can be successfully applied and removed. Of note, the terms insertion and application can be used interchangeably, however, more recently, there is a trend toward using the term "application" for scleral lenses. The application and removal process are heavily dependent on the cooperativity of the patient and compliance of the parent or caregiver. In this subsection, the parent or legal guardian will be referenced with the term caregiver. If cooperativity or compliance is at issue, then contact lenses are not a realistic option. The degree of cooperativity to contact lens wear is not necessarily determined only by age of the patient, as there are reports in literature of contact lenses being used in infants as young as a few weeks to months of age. In rare cases, when necessary, the application and removal of contact lenses can be performed under anesthesia for therapeutic, diagnostic, or fitting purposes. Murphy et al. demonstrated in their case report that for some patients unable to wear scleral lenses in the beginning, practitioners could start with a soft contact lens [78]. Once the patient is comfortable in wearing soft contact lenses, then he or she can transition to a piggyback soft contact lens-scleral lens system, then ultimately to a scleral lens alone. This transition helps some patients adapt to contact lens wear in order to ultimately achieve confidence with the scleral lens application and removal process.

Techniques

There are several techniques practitioners can employ to help pediatric patients and caregivers achieve successful application and removal of their contact lenses. Ultimately, all involved must consider the many options for approaching application and removal in order to achieve success, including; will the patient or caregiver be applying/removing the lenses, will the patient be more comfortable standing up, sitting down, or laying down over a bench. An alternate method for application of a scleral lens would be to have the patient lie across the caregiver's lap, the caregiver will hold the child's head and the practitioner will hold the lids and apply the lens at the same time. This method works best with two individuals but can be done alone if the child is cooperative or small enough to be swaddled. Being flexible in your approach and adapting to the patient's needs is essential. For pediatric patients with normal corneal sensation, the use of in-office proparacaine may be considered for the initial insertion of the lens, such as in a case of a pediatric corneal abrasion, however, proparacaine is absolutely contraindicated for at home use due to the risk of corneal melt.

For scleral lens application, since the bowl of the lens is filled with preservative-free normal saline solution, the patient's head must be positioned parallel to the floor. One technique to help with scleral lens application is using preservative-free gel or preservative-free ointment instead of saline to fill the bowl of the lens. These thicker solutions allow the patient to have more room for error when applying the lens without spilling the lens bowl solution. Additionally, these thicker solutions afford the option to insert the lens in a patient in the supine position. Families can slowly transition from ointment to saline use over the course of several months as the patient and caregiver get more comfortable with the process.

Application and removal technique for patients with normal corneal sensation and patients with neurotrophic corneas are different. The preservative-free normal saline solutions can feel cold which can be alarming for patients with normal corneal sensation. These solutions can be gently warmed by rolling the vial back and forth between the palm of the hands. Some pediatric patients are more successful with a gradual stepwise process. For example, starting the application training process by simply holding the fluid-filled lens just in contact with the cornea without attempting application can be a beneficial first step.

Time Commitment

The patient and caregiver(s) should be educated on the time commitment required for either the bandage contact lens or scleral lens fitting process, including not only the application and removal training, but also the predicted number of visits needed to achieve fit optimization and for proper follow-up care. For instance, the scleral lens treatment process can include several hours to learn proper techniques for application and removal and several visits to finalize the fit [21]. It is important to educate the patient and their caregiver(s) in order to set realistic expectations.

Additionally, this helps to ensure that the patient and caregiver(s) will not become discouraged if they do not successfully insert and remove the contact lens within their first few attempts. As well, practitioners and clinicians must be equally committed to the necessary time commitment, allowing for significantly more time for these patient visits within their busy clinic schedule. Walline et al. looked at the overall chair time for healthy pediatric patients initiating use of soft contact lenses [79]. The study found that total chair time took 15 min more for children (8–12 years old) vs teens (13–17 years old). The fitting time was the same for both age groups, but insertion and removal training took longer for children compared to teens. Currently, there is no literature reporting on scleral lens fitting time commitments for pediatric patients with ocular surface disease.

Some families may travel great distances to come for the office visits. It is important to educate these families especially on the expected number of visits for the entire bandage contact lens or scleral lens treatment process. Additionally, it can be helpful for some families to find a practitioner closer to home to help with minor concerns that may arise throughout the treatment process.

Training Family Members

Practitioners must determine who should be trained in the insertion and removal of the contact or scleral lens for the pediatric patient. The caregiver bringing the child into the exam may not be the individual who is always involved in the morning or bedtime routine, such as in instances of separation or divorce. If this social dynamic is not identified, the child may end up only wearing their lens periodically when they are with the trained caregiver. It is not uncommon to need to train several caregivers. For instance, frequently both parents work and another caregiver is responsible for the child throughout the day. This individual should also be educated on how to handle the lens if any issues arise. Additionally, there may be some caregivers that are more comfortable working with eyes (perhaps wears contact lenses themselves), who may be more successful at the application and removal process.

For school aged children, having contact lens supplies, such as a plunger and scleral lens solutions, with them at school is important. Often times, this responsibility can be undertaken by a school nurse. It is essential to inform and educate the school, including the patient's teacher and nurse, of their condition and provide them a basic understanding of lens handling and management.

Psychological Aspects of Insertion and Removal Training

Insertion and removal of bandage contact lenses and scleral lenses can initially be a frightening experience for children. From the child's perspective, the experience of a new person who is larger and stronger than them trying to touch their eyes can be vulnerable and scary, especially if they are already in pain. In the lens fitting and application and removal training process, it is of the utmost importance to be extremely patient, take your time and utilize breaks as needed. Being cognizant of the need to end the day's appointment and regroup at the next follow-up visit is vital. Throughout the visits explain to the family and patient what you are doing in order to try to make the child feel as comfortable as possible. In cases where cooperativity is more challenging, several visits of just talking, watching instructional videos, or holding the lens independently can be beneficial. Other room distractions such as animated videos or exciting fixation targets can as well play a role.

Socioeconomic

The cost of the lenses and additional costs associated with routine maintenance and lens care can be high. Families must consider these costs when committing to lens wear, including that it may be required to take time off work to come to the office visits. When applicable, caregivers should investigate if support services are available from their state or other eye care organizations.

Amblyopia

Chronic ocular surface irritation can lead to inflammation, which in time can result in scarring and decreased vision secondary to the physical opacity itself or irregular astigmatism. Depending on the patient's age, the potential for amblyopia must be taken into consideration. Corneal scarring can result in not only deprivational amblyopia but also refractive amblyopia potentially causing irreversible degradation of best corrected visual acuity. Therefore, timely contact lens fitting to manage ocular surface disease can ultimately play a secondary role in reducing the risk of amblyogenic pathology or rehabilitating vision that has reached an amblyogenic stage. Contact lens usage in these cases should be co-managed with the pediatric optometrist or ophthalmologist leading the amblyopia care to ensure any additional strategies, such as patching are integrated into the overall management plan.

Conclusion

Bandage contact lenses and scleral lenses are frequently reserved as management options for only adult patients. However, these treatment modalities can play an important role and provide an additional management strategy for acute and chronic ocular surface disease in pediatric eye care. This chapter has highlighted not only contact lens and scleral lens treatment options and indications for use, but also the many special considerations that must be addressed to successfully utilize these lenses in the management of pediatric ocular surface diseases.

References

1. Villani E, Nucci P. Pediatric dry eye. In: Knights Templar Eye Foundation Pediatric Ophthalmology Education. 2020. https://www.aao.org/disease-review/pediatric-dry-eye. Accessed 24 May 2022.
2. Moon JH, Kim KW, Moon NJ. Smartphone use is a risk factor for pediatric dry eye disease according to region and age: a case control study. BMC Ophthalmol. 2016;16:188.
3. Daniel MC, O'Gallagher M, Hingorani M, Dahlmann-Noor A, Tuft S. Challenges in the management of pediatric blepharokeratoconjunctivis/ocular rosacea. Expert Rev Ophthalmol. 2016;11:299–309.
4. Kamal SM, Riccobono K, Kwok A, Edmond JC, Pflugfelder SC. Unilateral pediatric neurotrophic keratitis due to congenital left trigeminal nerve aplasia with PROSE (prosthetic replacement of the ocular surface ecosystem) treatment. Am J Ophthalmol Case Rep. 2020;20:100854.
5. Remington CD, Jacobs DS. PROSE treatment for pediatric patients with neurotrophic keratitis. Invest Ophthalmol Vis Sci. 2015;56:6076.
6. Mantelli F, Nardella C, Tiberi E, Sacchetti M, Bruscolini A, Lambiase A. Congenital corneal anesthesia and neurotrophic keratitis: diagnosis and management. Biomed Res Int. 2015;2015:1.
7. Rojas-Carabali W, Uribe-Reina P, Muñoz-Ortiz J, et al. High prevalence of abnormal ocular surface tests in a healthy pediatric population. Clin Ophthalmol. 2020;14:3427–38.
8. Kaufman LB, Colby KA, Jacobs DS, Nischal KK, Pflugfelder SC. Are we missing dry eye in children? EyeNet Magazine; 2022.
9. Craig JP, Nelson JD, Azar DT, et al. TFOS DEWS II report executive summary. Ocul Surf. 2017;15:802–12.
10. Stapleton F, Alves M, Bunya VY, et al. TFOS DEWS II epidemiology report. Ocul Surf. 2017;15:334–65.
11. Allergan. Restasis (cyclosporine) ophthalmic prescribing label. 2012.
12. Stason WB, Razavi M, Jacobs DS, Shepard DS, Suaya JA, Johns L, Rosenthal P. Clinical benefits of the Boston ocular surface prosthesis. Am J Ophthalmol. 2010;149:54–61.
13. Agranat JS, Kitos NR, Jacobs DS. Prosthetic replacement of the ocular surface ecosystem: impact at 5 years. Br J Ophthalmol. 2016;100:1171–5.
14. Bennett ES. Contemporary scleral lenses: theory and application. Optom Vis Sci. 2018;95:687.
15. Weiner G, Jacobs DS, Mian SI, Patel S, v. Update on scleral lenses. EyeNet Magazine. 2018:27–9.
16. Bennett ES. GP and custom soft annual report 2021. Contact Lens Spectrum. 2021;36:20–7.
17. Hashim Thiab H. The evaluation of bandage soft contact lenses as a primary treatment for traumatic corneal abrasions. Int J Clin Experiment Ophthalmol. 2020;4:041–8.
18. Morrison R, Shovlin JP. A review of the use of bandage lenses. Metab Pediatr Syst Ophthalmol. 1982;6:117–21.
19. Bendoriene J, Vogt U. Therapeutic use of silicone hydrogel contact lenses in children. Eye Contact Lens. 2006;32:104–8.
20. Severinsky B, Lenhart P. Scleral contact lenses in the pediatric population-indications and outcomes. Cont Lens Anterior Eye. 2022;45:101452.
21. Rathi VM, Mandathara PS, Vaddavalli PK, Srikanth D, Sangwan VS. Fluid filled scleral contact lens in pediatric patients: challenges and outcome. Contact Lens Anterior Eye. 2012;35:189–92.
22. Gungor İ, Schor K, Rosenthal P, Jacobs DS. The Boston scleral lens in the treatment of pediatric patients. J AAPOS. 2008;12:263–7.

23. Jacobs DS, Carrasquillo KG, Cottrell PD, et al. CLEAR-medical use of contact lenses. Cont Lens Anterior Eye. 2021;44:289–329.
24. Jones L, Downie LE, Korb D, et al. TFOS DEWS II management and therapy report. Ocul Surf. 2017;15:575–628.
25. Goyal S, Hamrah P. Understanding neuropathic corneal pain—gaps and current therapeutic approaches. Semin Ophthalmol. 2016;31:59–70.
26. Galor A, Levitt RC, Felix ER, Martin ER, Sarantopoulos CD. Neuropathic ocular pain: an important yet underevaluated feature of dry eye. Eye. 2015;29:301–12.
27. Russo PA, Bouchard CS, Galasso JM. Extended-Wear silicone hydrogel soft contact lenses in the Management of Moderate to severe dry eye signs and symptoms secondary to graft-versus-host disease. Eye Contact Lens. 2007;33:144–7.
28. Lim L, Lim EWL. Therapeutic contact lenses in the treatment of corneal and ocular surface diseases—a review. Asia Pac J Ophthalmol. 2020;9:524–32.
29. de Brabander J, Kok JHC, Nuijts RMMA, Wenniger-Prick LJJM. A practical approach to and long-term results of fitting silicone contact lenses in aphakic children after congenital cataract. CLAO J. 2002;28:31–5.
30. Holden BA, Mertz GW. Critical oxygen levels to avoid corneal edema for daily and extended wear contact lenses. Invest Ophthalmol Vis Sci. 1984;25:1161–7.
31. Stapleton F, Keay L, Edwards K, Naduvilath T, Dart JKG, Brian G, Holden BA. The incidence of contact lens-related microbial keratitis in Australia. Ophthalmology. 2008;115:1655–62.
32. Bausch & Lomb Incorporated. Bausch & Lomb pure vision (balafilcon A) package insert/fitting guide. 2019:1–3.
33. Jacobs DS, Agranat JS. Therapeutic contact lenses in the Management of Corneal and Ocular Surface Disease. In: Foundations of corneal disease. Cham: Springer; 2020. p. 291–8.
34. Zambelli AM, Brothers KM, Hunt KM, Romanowski EG, Nau AC, Dhaliwal DK, Shanks RMQ. Diffusion of antimicrobials across silicone hydrogel contact lenses. Eye Contact Lens. 2015;41:277–80.
35. Chen L, Pi L, Ke N, Chen X, Liu Q. The protective efficacy and safety of bandage contact lenses in children aged 5 to 11 after frontalis muscle flap suspension for congenital blepharoptosis: a single-center randomized controlled trial. Medicine. 2017;96:e8003.
36. Sarac O, Caglayan M, Uysal BS, Uzel AGT, Tanriverdi B, Cagil N. Accelerated versus standard corneal collagen cross-linking in pediatric keratoconus patients: 24 months follow-up results. Contact Lens Anterior Eye. 2018;41:442–7.
37. Koçluk Y, Çetinkaya S, Alyamaç Sukgen E, Günay M, Mete A. Comparing the effects of two different contact lenses on corneal reepithelialization after corneal collagen cross-linking. Pak J Med Sci. 2017;33:680. https://doi.org/10.12669/pjms.333.12241.
38. Henriquez MA, Villegas S, Rincon M, Maldonado C, Izquierdo L. Long-term efficacy and safety after corneal collagen crosslinking in pediatric patients: three-year follow-up. Eur J Ophthalmol. 2018;28:415–8.
39. Liesegang TJ. Contact lens-related microbial keratitis: part I: epidemiology. Cornea. 1997;16:125–31.
40. Soleimani M, Tabatabaei SA, Mohammadi SS, Valipour N, Mirzaei A. A ten-year report of microbial keratitis in pediatric population under five years in a tertiary eye center. J Ophthalmic Inflamm Infect. 2020;10:35.
41. Barnett M, Courey C, Fadel D, et al. BCLA CLEAR-scleral lenses. Contact Lens Anterior Eye. 2021;44:270–88.
42. Rosenthal P, Cotter J. The Boston scleral lens in the management of severe ocular surface disease. Ophthalmol Clin N Am. 2003;16:89. https://doi.org/10.1016/S0896-1549(02)00067-6.
43. Shorter E, Schornack M, Harthan J, Nau A, Fogt J, Cao D, Nau C. Keratoconus patient satisfaction and care burden with corneal gas-permeable and scleral lenses. Optom Vis Sci. 2020;97:790–6.
44. Barnett M, Carrasquillo KG, Schornack MM. Clinical outcomes of scleral lens fitting with a data-driven, quadrant-specific design: multicenter review. Optom Vis Sci. 2020;97:761–5.

45. Perrson T. Material Management in a Scleral Society. Review of Cornea and Contact Lens. 2020.
46. Manning J. Making sense of scleral lens materials. Review of Cornea and Contact Lenses. 2018.
47. Boston Materials and Solutions Product guide. https://fit-boston.eu/downloads/pdf/ProductGuideEN.pdf. Accessed 27 Jul 2022.
48. Food and Drug Administration 510K summary, No K180988: Acuity 100 (hexafocon A) rigid gas permeable contact lens. https://www.accessdata.fda.gov/scripts/cdrh/cfdocs/cfpmn/pmn.cfm?ID=K180988. Accessed 27 Jul 2022.
49. Food and Drug Administration 510K summary, No K212631: Optimum infinite (tisilfocon A) daily wear contact lenses. https://www.accessdata.fda.gov/cdrh_docs/pdf21/K212631.pdf. Accessed 27 Jul 2022.
50. Food and Drug Administration 510K summary, No K103561: Menicon Z (tisilficon A) rigid gas permeable contact lens. https://www.accessdata.fda.gov/cdrh_docs/pdf10/K103561.pdf. Accessed 27 Jul 2022.
51. Food and Drug Administration 510K summary, No K203571: Acuity 200 (fluoroxyfocon A) rigid gas permeable contact lens. . https://www.accessdata.fda.gov/cdrh_docs/pdf20/K203571.pdf. Accessed 27 Jul 2022.
52. Jacobs DS, Rosenthal P. Boston scleral lens prosthetic device for treatment of severe dry eye in chronic graft-versus-host disease. Cornea. 2007;26:1195. https://doi.org/10.1097/ICO.0b013e318155743d.
53. Picot C, Gauthier AS, Campolmi N, Delbosc B. Quality of life in patients wearing scleral lenses. J Fr Ophtalmol. 2015;38:615–9.
54. Kreps EO, Pesudovs K, Claerhout I, Koppen C. Mini-scleral lenses improve vision-related quality of life in keratoconus. Cornea. 2021;40:859–64.
55. Baudin F, Chemaly A, Arnould L, Barrénéchea E, Lestable L, Bron AM, Creuzot-Garcher C. Quality-of-life improvement after scleral lens fitting in patients with keratoconus. Eye Contact Lens. 2021;47:520–5.
56. Ozek D, Kemer OE, Altiaylik P. Visual performance of scleral lenses and their impact on quality of life in patients with irregular corneas. Arq Bras Oftalmol. 2018;81:475–80.
57. Bhattacharya P, Mahadevan R. Quality of life and handling experience with the PROSE device: an Indian scenario. Clin Exp Optom. 2017;100:710–7.
58. Bligdon SM, Colarusso BA, Ganjei AY, Kwok A, Luo ZK, Brocks D. Scleral lens and prosthetic replacement of the ocular surface ecosystem utilization in ocular graft-versus-host disease: a survey study. Clin Ophthalmol. 2021;15:4829–38.
59. Asghari B, Brocks D, Carrasquillo KG, Crowley E. OSDI outcomes based on patient demographic and Wear patterns in prosthetic replacement of the ocular surface ecosystem. Clin Optom (Auckl). 2022;14:1–12.
60. Kok JHC, Visser R. Treatment of ocular surface disorders and dry eyes with high gas-permeable scleral lenses. Cornea. 1992;11:518–22.
61. Foss AJ, Trodd TC, Dart JK. Current indications for scleral contact lenses. CLAO J. 1994;20:115–8.
62. Tan DTH, Pullum KW, Buckley RJ. Medical applications of scleral contact lenses: 1. A retrospective analysis of 343 cases. Cornea. 1995;14:121–9.
63. Tan DTH, Pullum KW, Buckley RJ. Medical applications of scleral contact lenses: 2. Gas-permeable scleral contact lenses. Cornea. 1995;14:130–7.
64. Pullum K, Buckley R. A study of 530 patients referred for rigid gas permeable scleral contact lens assessment. Cornea. 1997;16:612–22.
65. Segal O, Barkana Y, Hourovitz D, Behrman S, Kamun Y, Avni I, Zadok D. Scleral contact lenses may help where other modalities fail. Cornea. 2003;22:308–10.
66. Pullum KW, Whiting MA, Buckley RJ. Scleral contact lenses: the expanding role. Cornea. 2005;24:269–77.
67. Rosenthal P, Croteau A. Fluid-ventilated, gas-permeable scleral contact lens is an effective option for managing severe ocular surface disease and many corneal disorders that would otherwise require penetrating keratoplasty. Eye Contact Lens. 2005;31:130–4.

68. Severinsky B, Lenhart P. Scleral contact lenses in the pediatric population-indications and outcomes. Cont Lens Anterior Eye. 2021;44:19. https://doi.org/10.1016/J.CLAE.2021.101452.
69. Rathi VM, Mandathara PS, Vaddavalli K, Srikanth D, Sangwan VS. Fluid filled scleral contact lens in pediatric patients: challenges and outcome. Cont Lens Anterior Eye. 2012;35:189–92.
70. Alipour F, Jamshidi Gohari S, Azad N, Mehrdad R. Miniscleral contact lens in pediatric age group: indications, safety, and efficacy. Eye Contact Lens. 2021;47:408–12.
71. Fuller DG, Wang Y. Safety and efficacy of scleral lenses for keratoconus. Optom Vis Sci. 2020;97:741–8.
72. Cressey A, Jacobs DS, Remington C, Carrasquillo KG. Improvement of chronic corneal opacity in ocular surface disease with prosthetic replacement of the ocular surface ecosystem (PROSE) treatment. Am J Ophthalmol Case Rep. 2018;10:108. https://doi.org/10.1016/j.ajoc.2018.02.010.
73. Liao J, Asghari B, Carrasquillo KG. Regression of corneal opacity and neovascularization in Stevens-Johnson syndrome and toxic epidermal necrolysis with the use of prosthetic replacement of the ocular surface ecosystem (PROSE) treatment. Am J Ophthalmol Case Rep. 2022;101520:101520.
74. Cressey A, Jacobs DS, Carrasquillo KG. Management of vascularized limbal keratitis with prosthetic replacement of the ocular surface system. Eye Contact Lens. 2012;38:137. https://doi.org/10.1097/ICL.0b013e31823bafbc.
75. Rosenthal P, Cotter J, Baum J. Treatment of persistent corneal epithelial defect with extended Wear of a fluid-ventilated gas-permeable scleral contact lens. Am J Ophthalmol. 2000;130:33. https://doi.org/10.1016/S0002-9394(00)00379-2.
76. Lim P, Ridges R, Jacobs DS, Rosenthal P. Treatment of persistent corneal epithelial defect with overnight wear of a prosthetic device for the ocular surface. Am J Ophthalmol. 2013;156:1095. https://doi.org/10.1016/j.ajo.2013.06.006.
77. Ciralsky JB, Chapman KO, Rosenblatt MI, Sood P, Fernandez AGA, Lee MN, Sippel KC. Treatment of refractory persistent corneal epithelial defects: a standardized approach using continuous Wear PROSE therapy. Ocul Immunol Inflamm. 2015;23:219–24.
78. Murphy DA, Samples JS, Zepeda EM, Riaz KM. Progression from soft lens to piggyback soft-scleral contact lens system to facilitate scleral lens use in a pediatric patient. Eye Contact Lens. 2021;47:426–8.
79. Walline JJ, Jones LA, Rah MJ, Manny RE, Berntsen DA, Chitkara M, Gaume A, Kim A, Quinn N, CLIP STUDY GROUP. Contact lenses in pediatrics (CLIP) study: chair time and ocular health. Optom Vis Sci. 2007;84:896–902.

Chapter 10
Surgical Rehabilitation of the Ocular Surface in Children

Adanna Udeh and Christina Prescott

Introduction

Corneal lesions or opacities in the pediatric population are important causes of vision loss as they can lead to amblyopia from induced astigmatism or sensory deprivation. In rare circumstances, surgical intervention is indicated to optimize the ocular surface and preserve visual function. Etiologies can vary from relatively common causes such as phlyctenular and blepharoconjunctivitis disease to rarer causes such as infectious, congenital, or neoplastic disease. Surgical interventions in the pediatric population require extensive planning, often including preoperative exams under anesthesia and coordination with multidisciplinary teams. Furthermore, it is important to realize that the efficacy of an intervention relies heavily on diligent postoperative management, and in many circumstances, amblyopia may still limit the visual potential. Hence, detailed and extensive discussions with the primary caregivers are critical to review expectations for appropriate follow-up, signs of complications, and need for urgent re-evaluation. In some situations, educating caregivers to perform a preliminary external eye exam with a penlight may be beneficial. This chapter will discuss indications, techniques, and postoperative care for specific surgical interventions including tarsorrhaphy, corneal gluing, phototherapeutic keratectomy, surgical removal of lesions, amniotic membrane grafting, corneal patch grafts, limbal stem cell transplantation, and corneal neurotization.

A. Udeh · C. Prescott (✉)
Department of Ophthalmology, NYU Langone Health, Grossman School of Medicine, New York, NY, USA
e-mail: Adanna.udeh@nyulangone.org; Christina.prescott@nyulangone.org

© The Author(s), under exclusive license to Springer Nature Switzerland AG 2023
A. Traish, V. P. Douglas (eds.), *Pediatric Ocular Surface Disease*,
https://doi.org/10.1007/978-3-031-30562-7_10

Tarsorrhaphy

Indication

A tarsorrhaphy creates a mechanical closure of the eyelid, with the apposition of mucosal membranes. Tarsorrhaphy can be done primarily or following a primary surgical intervention, including a lesion removal, amniotic membrane, or patch graft. Eyelid closure promotes epithelial healing by decreasing the evaporation of tears, thus keeping the tear film layer intact to maintain the ocular surface [1]. Indications for a primary procedure include persistent epithelial defects as seen in neurotrophic keratitis and diseases resulting in exposure, such as facial nerve palsy or congenital globe dystopia with exophthalmos. Occlusive measures must be used judiciously in the pediatric population given the risk of sensory deprivation amblyopia.

Surgical Techniques

Temporary

- Simple suture: A simple suture can be either a mattress suture with or without a bolster or serpentine suture. In both circumstances, the suture is run between the gray line (the muscle of Riolan) of the upper and lower eyelid, and out through the eyelid skin. The free suture ends can be secured by steri-strips to the upper eyelid (in simple stitch) or lateral and medial canthal skin (serpentine) to allow for tightness adjustment for examination or to ensure corneal protection. Depending on the suture type (6-0 prolene/6-0 Vicryl/4-0 silk), this technique may be secure for several weeks (Fig. 10.1).
- Cyanoacrylate placement for temporary closure: The use of cyanoacrylate adhesive can also be used for temporary closure [2] and can be done in-office or after another surgical procedure under anesthesia. With this technique, the adhesive is applied directly to the eyelid margin while the eyelids are held closed.

Permanent

- Reversible margin annealing tarsorrhaphy: When needed for more than a few weeks, the eyelid margins are denuded and the epithelium is then sewn together to create an attachment.
- Permanent: A segment of the upper tarsus is transported with a segment of the upper eyelid. This is rarely done in children.

Postoperative Care and Complications

In the immediate postoperative period, an antibiotic topical ointment may be applied to the skin to prevent secondary infection of the suture sites. Follow-up frequency and the duration of the tarsorrhaphy depend on the indication for the procedure.

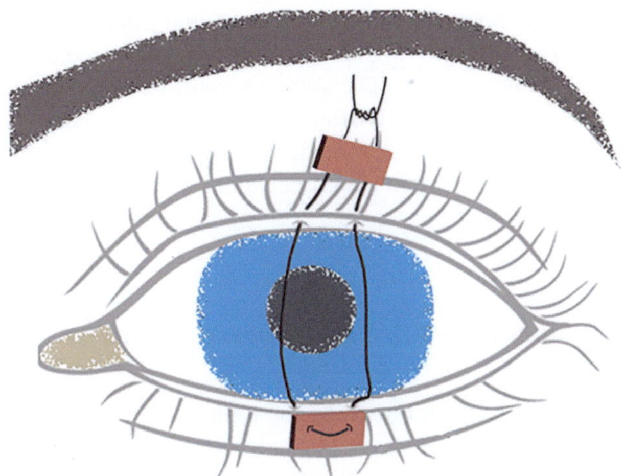

Fig. 10.1 Surgical diagram illustrating the simple suture tarsorrhaphy technique. Note the use of bolsters for skin protection and suture reinforcement

Sutures may be cut in the office or may be removed under sedation in the operating room depending on the age and cooperation of the patient.

Corneal Gluing

Indication

Cyanoacrylate adhesives are monomers, which rapidly polymerize and bond in the presence of water or weak bases, causing them to harden. As short-chain derivatives are strongest, N-butyl cyanoacrylate compounds are greater than octyl-cyanoacrylates. Cyanoacrylates are also bacteriostatic, particularly against gram-positive organisms including group A streptococci, *Streptococcus pneumoniae*, and *Staphylococcus aureus*. Similar to bond strength, the bacteriostatic quality increases with shorter chain derivatives [3]. The most common indications for cyanoacrylate glue are corneal ulcers, and corneal perforations less than 3 mm in diameter. Corneal lesions adjacent to the limbus are not good candidates for corneal gluing since the conjunctiva is not as adherent. The application of cyanoacrylate adhesive has been shown to interfere with stromal melting of both infective and non-infective etiologies and decreases the polymorphonuclear inflammatory activity [4].

Surgical Technique

In adult patients, glue application can be performed either at the slit lamp or in a minor procedure room. However, given the nature of the pediatric population and the inability to remain stationary for appropriate placement, an operating room setting is preferred for children. After placement of an eyelid speculum, the cornea should be debrided of necrotic tissue and dried. The cyanoacrylate adhesive can be drawn up into a syringe and placed over the corneal defect using a small gauge (27 or 30 gauge) needle. The adhesive must be applied quickly as it begins to dry and harden within seconds after placement. Other techniques of glue application have been described, which include placing the glue on a small piece of sterile drape and applying the drape to the corneal defect to provide a smooth border for BCL placement [5].

Postoperative Care and Complications

The main concern regarding the topical use of cyanoacrylate pertains to the potential toxic effect of direct contact with the cornea and anterior chamber. However, this may be difficult to discern as keratitis and anterior chamber inflammation may be part of the original disease processes necessitating corneal gluing. Hence, close follow-up is needed to monitor the progression of the microbial disease, especially in the setting of BCL use.

PTK (Phototherapeutic Keratectomy)

Indication

Phototherapeutic keratectomy, first performed in 1985 and approved by the FDA in 1995, can be used to treat pathology of the superficial cornea. It employs an excimer laser (ultraviolet light) to interrupt molecular bonds within the tissue in a low heat-generating process termed photoablation [6]. This process may present a less invasive alternative to procedures such as lamellar or penetrating keratoplasty, with faster visual rehabilitation and less activity restriction. In children, indications may include corneal dystrophies, post-traumatic/post-infectious scarring, band keratopathy, recurrent epithelial erosions, and other surface irregularities [7]. However, the corneal refractive changes induced by laser use must be considered before proceeding with laser therapy. In general, each pulse of the excimer laser removes approximately 0.25 μm of corneal tissue, with about 50 pulses producing approximately 1 diopter of hyperopic shift. These values may vary based on the degree or depth of the corneal pathology [8].

Surgical Technique

As stated previously, the requirements for sedation depend on the age and cooperation of the patient, and as with most pediatric procedures, general anesthesia is commonly used. Prior to beginning any laser surgery, the excimer laser must be calibrated, and the ablation zone diameter and ablation depth should be programmed and confirmed. A masking agent such as hydroxypropyl methylcellulose is frequently applied during the procedure to achieve a smooth ablation. Depending on the indication for ablation, manual debridement of the corneal surface may be needed before laser treatment. In other circumstances, lesions can be treated via a trans-epithelial approach, minimizing the necessity for a full-thickness corneal epithelial abrasion. At the termination of the case, a bandage contact lens is usually placed to reduce discomfort.

Postoperative Care and Complications

Close follow-up is needed, especially during the first postoperative month. The residual corneal thickness following PTK should be carefully considered to reduce the risk of ectasia. Further potential complications include sub-epithelial haze, which usually resolves within the first year postoperatively. Depending on the indication for treatment, there may be a risk of recurrence of the inciting pathology. Additionally, any resultant refractive changes will need to be addressed: PTK may be combined with or followed by PRK or refractive correction via contact lens or spectacles. Cycloplegic refraction is necessary in these children, due to the hyperopic effect of the laser. While laser refractive surgery in the pediatric population is still considered controversial, the literature has shown promising results as a viable treatment option for some children.

Surgical Removal of Lesion

Indication

Ocular surface lesions in the pediatric population are rare and can have multiple etiologies from inflammatory to neoplastic. When planning removal of a lesion, multiple factors (size, depth, cosmesis, and the risk of amblyopia) must be considered. While ocular surface tumors are rare in children overall, the most common growths are benign epibulbar dermoids. The techniques described here can be employed for most benign surface lesions; however, we will focus on limbal dermoid removal.

Epibulbar dermoids are the most common type of epibulbar tumor in the pediatric age group. They represent congenital growths of normal tissue (i.e., choristoma) and can vary widely in their presentation, but are most frequently located at the inferotemporal conjunctiva. Epibulbar dermoids can be classified into 3 grades, each with increasing degrees of anterior structure involvement [9]:

- Grade 1: Superficial lesions less than 5 mm localized to the limbus
- Grade 2: Lesions >5 mm, extending the depth of the cornea without involvement of Descemet's membrane
- Grade 3: Large lesions, covering the entirety of the cornea with extension through anterior segment structures between the corneal endothelium and pigmented iris epithelium

Clinical indications for surgical removal and reconstruction are indicated for grade 2 and 3 lesions given the high risk of amblyopia. In grade 1 lesions, resection may be considered to reduce amblyopia in patients unresponsive to conservative measures, patients with cosmetic concerns, or incomplete eyelid closure which can worsen corneal surface disease. A complete preoperative examination, under anesthesia, depending on the patient's age, with the use of topography or ultrasound biomicroscopy (UBM), may be needed to assist with surgical planning.

Surgical Techniques

Several surgical techniques have been described in the literature based on the size, depth, and site of the lesions [10].

- Superficial keratectomy: Small lesions that are superficial (limited to the corneal epithelium or anterior stroma) can be gently removed with the use of a diamond or crescent blade. A shallow defect may be closed with an amniotic membrane graft applied with fibrin glue (see Fig. 10.3 and section on amniotic membrane grafting in this chapter).
- Lamellar keratoplasty: When you are faced with deeper lesions with more stromal involvement, a lamellar patch graft can be measured to the corresponding defect using a trephine or skin punch biopsy tool, and secured to the lesion using 10-0 nylon or Vicryl sutures after the lesion is excised. Split thickness irradiated corneal tissue can be used for the graft to reduce the need for fresh corneal tissue. (please see Fig. 10.4 and section on corneal patch grafting in this chapter).

Postoperative Care and Complications

Caution should be taken intraoperatively to avoid globe rupture when resecting deeper lesions. Postoperative management requires frequent use of topical steroids and antibiotics to reduce inflammation and subsequent scarring because children mount a robust inflammatory response. A long topical steroid taper of several weeks to months may be warranted, depending on the degree of inflammation and vascularization.

Amniotic Membrane Grafting

Indication

The use of an amniotic membrane graft (AMG) was introduced in the 1940s for the treatment of ocular surface disorders. As a biological membrane, amniotic membrane can promote the healing and growth of epithelial cells. It has also been postulated to have anti-inflammatory effects, therefore decreasing scar formation through the inhibition of fibroblast activation and can act as a physical barrier to infection [11]. Amniotic membrane is primarily used in conjunctival disorders, persistent corneal defects, bullous keratopathy, and after symblepharon removal (ocular surface reconstruction—as seen in inflammatory sequelae such as SJS and mucous membrane pemphigoid), and after thermal and chemical burns. The AMG can also be combined with other techniques to maximize epithelial healing [12].

Surgical Techniques

- Prokera is an alternative to AMG that can be placed into the eye similar to a large diameter, rigid contact lens. This is primarily used as a temporizing measure for children who cannot be brought to the operating room and who cannot have a surgical procedure performed at the bedside. These lenses are uncomfortable and may not fit well in the smaller eyes of children. Also, the amniotic membrane attached to these devices do not adequately cover the conjunctiva, so are best when the pathology is localized to the cornea.
- If the area of concern is localized to the cornea, the amniotic membrane is typically applied in two layers: one to cover the focal area of thinning and another to cover the surrounding cornea and promote healing. A small patch of amniotic membrane can be cut to fit the area of thinning and either glued or sutured in place. Then, a larger AMG is applied over the entire cornea and typically secured with perilimbal sutures to promote healing (Fig. 10.2).
- For patients with conjunctival involvement, such as in SJS, the entire conjunctiva and eyelid margin will need to be treated. There are multiple published techniques, using both glue and sutures to attach the membrane, and the technique can be modified based on the areas that needs to be covered [13]. Typically, the AMG should be placed onto the eyelid skin and fixated to the eyelid margin with 8-0 nylon suture. The AMG can then be spread epithelial side down to cover the entire cornea and conjunctival membrane. The AMG can be secured into the fornix by either passing a 6-0 prolene suture as deep into the fornices as possible (this can be done nasally and temporally for both the upper the lower lid) and sutured to the eyelid skin, or a symblepharon ring can be used to maintain the fornices. The AMG can be secured to the conjunctiva with 10-0 Vicryl sutures at each quadrant approximately 2 mm posterior to the limbus (Fig. 10.3).

- Depending on the underlying etiology, it is often beneficial to place a temporary tarsorrhaphy following the AMG procedure to promote healing.

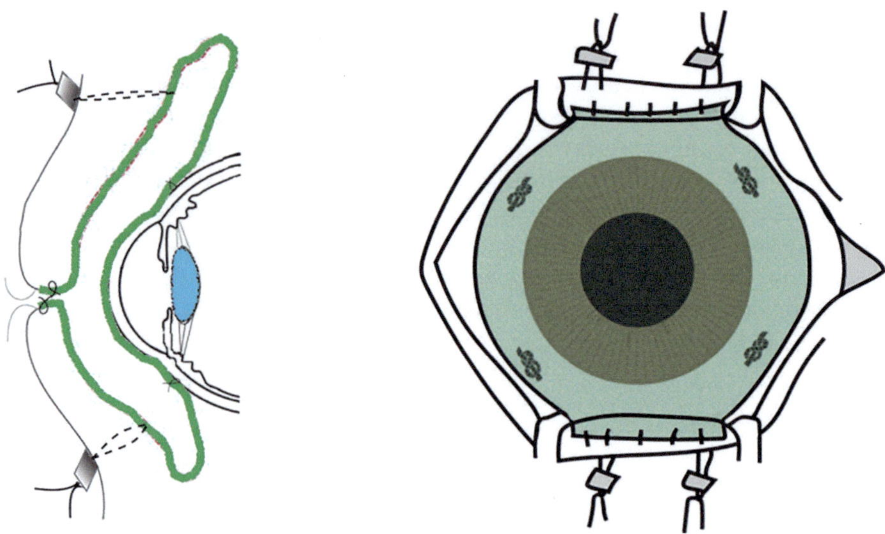

Fig. 10.2 Surgical technique demonstrating use of bilayer amniotic membrane. The first layer is sutured to the cornea directly over the defect, with a larger amniotic membrane then placed over the entire cornea and sutured to the perilimbal conjunctival and episclera

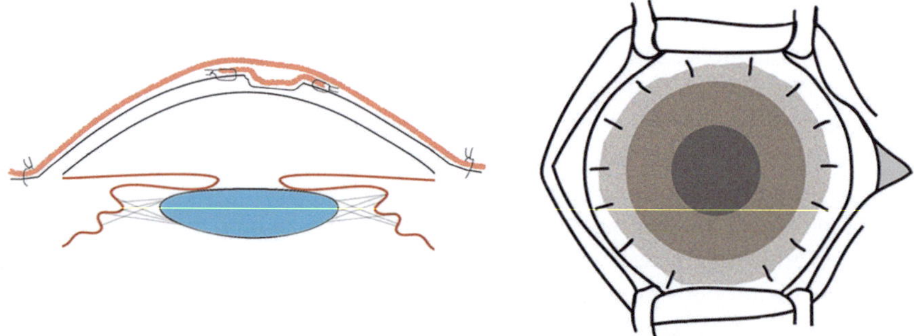

Fig. 10.3 Surgical technique demonstrating the amniotic membrane sutured to the perilimbal conjunctiva at each quadrant, with sutures passed deep into the fornices and sutured to the eyelid margin superiorly and inferiorly

Postoperative Care and Complications

In the pediatric population, the use of an ointment such as tobramycin-dexamethasone can be utilized both on the ocular surface and around the lid margins. The rate of amniotic membrane degradation depends on the severity of inflammation, and re-application should be considered in cases of severe inflammation. Few adverse reactions are reported overall and may include pyogenic granuloma from suture placement, hematoma beneath the graft, and postoperative infection.

Corneal Patch Graft

Indication

Corneal patch grafts can be utilized for corneal perforations, focal scarring, or thinning too small to warrant a full-size penetrating keratoplasty. Corneal patch grafts are indeed a form of transplantation, and since transplantation complication rates are much higher in the pediatric population, a careful preoperative examination and discussion must be had with all providers and caregivers involved. Any potential barriers to consistent postoperative follow-up and management would need to be carefully addressed to optimize outcomes [14]. A preoperative examination under anesthesia should be performed with imaging such as topography, ultrasound biomicroscopy, or anterior segment OCT to guide surgical planning. The etiology of corneal disease requiring a patch graft can be classified into congenital (i.e., limbal dermoids—(Fig. 10.4)), acquired non-traumatic (scarring most often secondary to microbial or viral keratitis), and acquired traumatic and varies with the age of the child and across geographic regions.

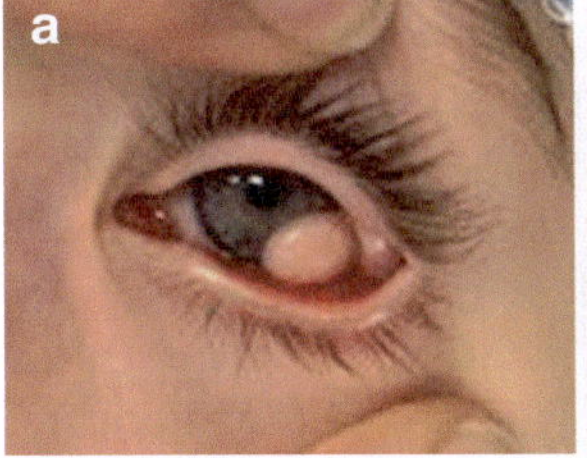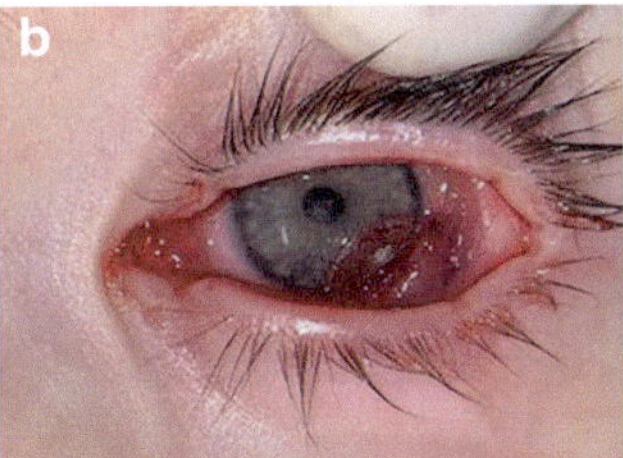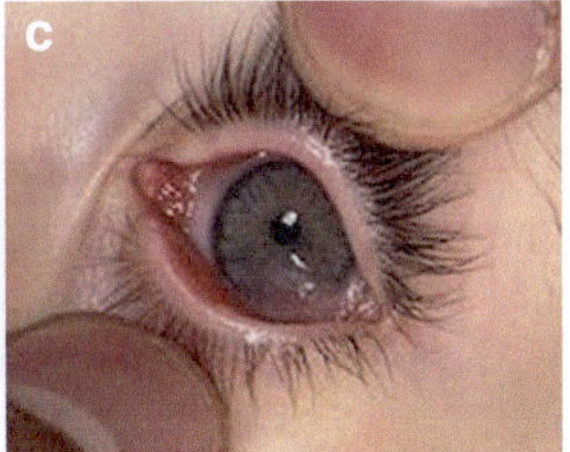

Fig. 10.4 (**a**) Pediatric patient with a limbal dermoid of the left eye. (**b**) Patient immediately following removal of the lesion with a lamellar corneal patch graft. (**c**) Patient at 6 months after surgery. Images obtained from personal archive of author CP

Surgical Technique

Corneal patch grafts may be lamellar or full thickness. With the patient under general anesthesia, the corneal lesion should be measured and an appropriate-sized trephine or skin biopsy punch is then used to outline and remove the affected corneal tissue with aid of a bent crescent blade. The residual defect is then re-measured. The patch graft is measured and prepared with a graft-host disparity of 0.25–0.5 mm, with the graft being oversized relative to the host cornea defect. The graft is secured to the lesion with 10-0 nylon sutures, and a bandage lens can sometimes be placed for comfort. Alternatively, a temporary tarsorrhaphy may be used to promote healing during the postoperative period [15].

Post-op Care and Complications

Early on daily to weekly follow-up is needed for close monitoring in the immediate postoperative period. As children tend to mount a strong inflammatory response, topical steroids should be administered frequently and tapered slowly. Additionally, early suture removal (within the first month) can be considered given the high risk of corneal neovascularization in the pediatric population. Complication rates are higher in this population and include infection, prolonged inflammation, graft rejection, trauma, glaucoma, and graft-host junction dehiscence.

Limbal Stem Cell Transplantation

Indication

The limbus functions as a reservoir of stem cells, contained in the palisades of Vogt, to support the corneal epithelium after infectious, inflammatory, or traumatic insults. Damage to the limbal stem cells can lead to loss of corneal transparency and subsequent vision loss. Transplantation of limbal stem cells was introduced in the 1980s and has led to successful regeneration of the ocular surface in select patients [16]. In the pediatric population, limbal stem cell deficiency (LSCD) can occur in the setting of multiple etiologies such as Steven Johnson syndrome, following ocular trauma including thermal or alkali injuries, and after infections such as herpetic keratitis. These eyes may have additional ocular pathology, including glaucoma, which can also affect visual potential.

The use of limbal stem cell transplants, especially in children, provides a treatment conundrum that must be carefully evaluated on a case-by-case basis. On the one hand, early intervention during the disease process will significantly increase the risk of graft failure. Alternatively, the risk of amblyopia, be it deprivation from corneal vascularization and scarring or refractive from induced irregular astigmatism can be high [17]. In cases of bilateral limbal stem cell deficiency, there is the additional consideration of lifelong immunosuppression following transplantation from a donor. In cases of unilateral limbal stem cell deficiency, the visual potential of the affected eye must be weighed against the risk of any surgical intervention to the unaffected eye.

Surgical Techniques

The surgical approach depends on whether the pathology is bilateral or unilateral, and if the entire limbus is affected.

- Autograft: Using tissue from the contralateral healthy eye (cultured or direct) [18].
- Cultured limbal epithelial transplantation (CLET): Primarily developed to minimize the drawbacks of whole tissue transplantation, namely needing 3–6 clock hours of tissue, which potentially induces LSCD in the donor eye. It begins with the laboratory culture of limbal epithelial cells where a small piece of healthy limbal tissue (less than one clock hour) is expanded within a culture media. Because only small amounts of donor tissue are needed, the process can be repeated in the event of an initial failure with minimal risk of adverse reaction to the donor's eye. The interval between repeat CLET can vary from 3–12 months. Additionally, CLET can be done sequentially, preceding keratoplasty with improved corneal graft survival reported in the literature.
- Simple limbal epithelial transplantation (SLET): While CLET provides an effective and efficient way to stabilize the ocular surface, it is not without significant drawbacks. The extensive cost for properly trained technicians/culture specialists, appropriate laboratory equipment, culture media, and facility fees make this option unfeasible for many patients as well as hospital systems. SLET minimizes these drawbacks while demonstrating similar ocular surface outcomes. In SLET, a small limbal biopsy of approximately 2×2 mm is retrieved from the healthy eye. The specimen is then cut into small pieces and attached to the amniotic membrane graft using fibrin glue. This apparatus is then attached to the recipient eye, allowing the limbal epithelial cells to culture in situ.
- Allogeneic donor (allograft): Can also be cultivated or direct. However allogenic transplantation has a high rejection rate and requires long-term immunosuppression so is not commonly performed in children [19].

Postoperative Care and Complications

A contact lens can be placed after the procedure to minimize trauma to the grafts. Frequent examinations are necessary within the first month postoperatively for close monitoring of the healing process. Frequent administration of both topical antibiotics and steroids is needed along with frequent ocular lubrication to promote epithelial healing.

Corneal Neurotization

Indication

Neurotrophic keratopathy (NK) in the pediatric population is challenging to diagnose and manage, due to the difficulty of the pediatric exam as well as the variability (or frequent absence) of pediatric subjective complaints. Corneal innervation is primarily obtained from the ophthalmic branch of the trigeminal nerve and controls reflex tearing and blinking which is critical for the maintenance of corneal epithelial and limbal stem cell health and function. Poor sensation can lead to chronic corneal epithelial defects, ulceration, and ultimately perforation and scarring [20]. Traditional therapeutic modalities have included tarsorrhaphy, pharmacologic ptosis, amniotic membrane grafting, and Gunderson flaps which all risk deprivation amblyopia in the pediatric population. Corneal neurotization is a newer technique that allows restoration of corneal sensation by re-forming neural pathways between the cornea and a healthy branch of the trigeminal nerve [21]. Improved corneal sensation helps maintain the stromal and epithelial integrity and clarity and reduces the rejection rate of subsequent keratoplasty. Neurotrophic keratopathy can occur for multiple reasons. More common causes are infections such as viral keratitis (herpes simplex), chemical burns, or injuries. More rare causes include intracranial lesions that may compress the trigeminal nerve along its tract, dysautonomia, Goldenhar syndrome with trigeminal aplasia, and familial trigeminal anesthesia.

Surgical Technique

This surgical technique involves connecting the cornea to a healthy ipsilateral or contralateral trigeminal nerve, a process termed "direct communication," or using an interposition (autologous or allogenic graft) also termed "indirect communication" (Fig. 10.5):

- Direct: In the direct technique, the donor nerve is mobilized from surrounding tissue, tunneled to the limbus, and secured directly onto the cornea. The use of both the supratrochlear and supraorbital nerves has been described with the use of a hemicoronal or bicoronal incision [22].
- Indirect: In this technique, an allogeneic or autologous nerve graft (most commonly the sural nerve, however, the lateral antebrachial cutaneous nerve and greater surgical nerve have been described) can be used to connect the donor graft through the subconjunctival space to the corneoscleral junction [23].

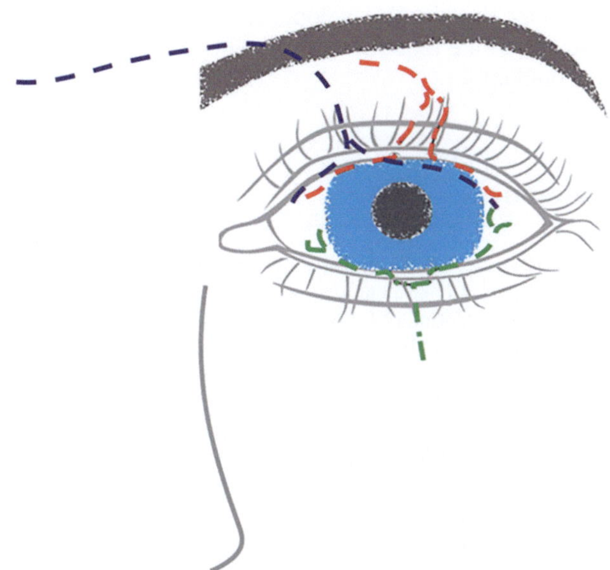

Fig. 10.5 Surgical techniques of corneal neurotization. A nerve graft (blue) can be used to anastomose the contralateral supratrochlear nerve or supraorbital nerve. The ipsilateral supratrochlear (red) or infraorbital (green) nerve can be directly attached to the limbus

Postoperative Care and Complications

Close follow-up is needed in the acute postoperative phase while the corneal epithelium and graft connections heal. Use of topical antibiotics and steroids is frequently employed. Depending on the age of the patient, a tarsorrhaphy may be needed to ensure protection and healing of the operative site. There are several methods to measure the corneal sensation, including using an esthesiometer, or a wisp of cotton. Successful restoration of corneal sensation can also be assessed clinically by improvement of the ocular surface including improved corneal clarity, decreased corneal fluorescein staining, and decreased corneal vascularization. The postoperative time to reestablish corneal sensation can range from 2 to 12 months and depends on the degree of neurotrophic keratopathy and the health of the donor nerve and graft.

Conclusion

Over recent years, several techniques have been developed or modified for use in the pediatric population to optimize the ocular surface. While their indications vary widely, they share a common rule: surgical intervention is rare and should be considered on a case-by-case basis. Additionally, given that any invasive intervention may alter the visual development of the pediatric patient, extensive and detailed discussions are required with all caregivers and providers involved to achieve optimal outcomes.

References

1. Acharya M, Gour A, Dave A. Commentary: Tarsorrhaphy: a stitch in time. Indian J OphthalmolIndian J Ophthalmol. 2020;68(1):33–4.
2. Trivedi D, McCalla M, Squires Z, Parulekar M. Use of cyanoacrylate glue for temporary tarsorrhaphy in children. Ophthalmic Plast Reconstr Surg. 2014;30(1):60–3.
3. Eiferman RA, Snyder JW. Antibacterial effect of cyanoacrylate glue. Arch Ophthalmol. 1983;101(6):958–60.
4. Deshmukh R, Stevenson LJ, Vajpayee R. Management of corneal perforations: an update. Indian J OphthalmolIndian J Ophthalmol. 2020;68(1):7–14.
5. Vote BJ, Elder MJ. Cyanoacrylate glue for corneal perforations: a description of a surgical technique and a review of the literature. Clin Exp Ophthalmol. 2000;28(6):437–42.
6. Kollias AN, Spitzlberger GM, Thurau S, Gruterich M, Lackerbauer CA. Phototherapeutic keratectomy in children. J Refract Surg. 2007;23(7):703–8.
7. Nagpal R, Maharana PK, Roop P, Murthy SI, Rapuano CJ, Titiyal JS, et al. Phototherapeutic keratectomy. Surv Ophthalmol. 2020;65(1):79–108.
8. Wilson SE, Marino GK, Medeiros CS, Santhiago MR. Phototherapeutic keratectomy: science and art. J Refract Surg. 2017;33(3):203–10.
9. Pirouzian A. Management of pediatric corneal limbal dermoids. Clin Ophthalmol. 2013;7:607–14.
10. Lang SJ, Bohringer D, Reinhard T. Surgical management of corneal limbal dermoids: retrospective study of different techniques and use of Mitomycin C. Eye (Lond). 2014;28(7):857–62.
11. Goyal R, Jones SM, Espinosa M, Green V, Nischal KK. Amniotic membrane transplantation in children with symblepharon and massive pannus. Arch Ophthalmol. 2006;124(10):1435–40.
12. Ahmad MS, Frank GS, Hink EM, Palestine AG, Gregory DG, McCourt EA. Amniotic membrane transplants in the pediatric population. J AAPOS. 2017;21(3):215–8.
13. Gregory DG. USA: ophthalmologic evaluation and management of acute Stevens-Johnson syndrome. Front Med (Lausanne). 2021;8:670643.
14. Zhu AY, Marquezan MC, Kraus CL, Prescott CR. Pediatric corneal transplants: review of current practice patterns. Cornea. 2018;37(8):973–80.
15. Sharma S, Rathi A, Murthy SI, Trivedi M, Patel C, Mohamed A, et al. Outcomes of penetrating and lamellar corneal patch grafts. Cornea. 2021;40(5):618–23.
16. Thoft RA. Keratoepithelioplasty. Am J Ophthalmol. 1984;97(1):1–6.
17. Choi SH, Kim MK, Oh JY. Corneal Limbal stem cell deficiency in children with Stevens-Johnson syndrome. Am J Ophthalmol. 2019;199:1–8.
18. Ramachandran C, Basu S, Sangwan VS, Balasubramanian D. Concise review: the coming of age of stem cell treatment for corneal surface damage. Stem Cells Transl Med. 2014;3(10):1160–8.
19. Atallah MR, Palioura S, Perez VL, Amescua G. Limbal stem cell transplantation: current perspectives. Clin Ophthalmol. 2016;10:593–602.
20. Ting DSJ, Figueiredo GS, Henein C, Barnes E, Ahmed O, Mudhar HS, et al. Corneal Neurotization for neurotrophic keratopathy: clinical outcomes and in vivo confocal microscopic and histopathological findings. Cornea. 2018;37(5):641–6.
21. Solyman O, Elhusseiny AM, Ali SF, Allen R. A review of pediatric corneal Neurotization. Int Ophthalmol Clin. 2022;62(1):83–94.
22. Terzis JK, Dryer MM, Bodner BI. Corneal neurotization: a novel solution to neurotrophic keratopathy. Plast Reconstr Surg. 2009;123(1):112–20.

23. Elbaz U, Bains R, Zuker RM, Borschel GH, Ali A. Restoration of corneal sensation with regional nerve transfers and nerve grafts: a new approach to a difficult problem. JAMA Ophthalmol. 2014;132(11):1289–95.
24. Dua HS, Azuara-Blanco A. Amniotic membrane transplantation. Br J Ophthalmol. 1999;83(6):748–52.
25. Ahmad S. Concise review: limbal stem cell deficiency, dysfunction, and distress. Stem Cells Transl Med. 2012;1(2):110–5.
26. Autrata R, Rehurek J, Vodickova K. Phototherapeutic keratectomy in children: 5-year results. J Cataract Refract Surg. 2004;30(9):1909–16.
27. Basu S, Mohamed A, Chaurasia S, Sejpal K, Vemuganti GK, Sangwan VS. Clinical outcomes of penetrating keratoplasty after autologous cultivated limbal epithelial transplantation for ocular surface burns. Am J Ophthalmol. 2011;152(6):917–24 e1.
28. Han ES, Wee WR, Lee JH, Kim MK. Long-term outcome and prognostic factor analysis for keratolimbal allografts. Graefes Arch Clin Exp Ophthalmol. 2011;249(11):1697–704.
29. Le Q, Chauhan T, Yung M, Tseng CH, Deng SX. Outcomes of Limbal stem cell transplant: a meta-analysis. JAMA Ophthalmol. 2020;138(6):660–70.
30. Rathi VM, Vyas SP, Vaddavalli PK, Sangwan VS, Murthy SI. Phototherapeutic keratectomy in pediatric patients in India. Cornea. 2010;29(10):1109–12.
31. Shanbhag SS, Patel CN, Goyal R, Donthineni PR, Singh V, Basu S. Simple limbal epithelial transplantation (SLET): review of indications, surgical technique, mechanism, outcomes, limitations, and impact. Indian J OphthalmolIndian J Ophthalmol. 2019;67(8):1265–77.
32. Tychsen L. Refractive surgery for special needs children. Arch Ophthalmol. 2009;127(6):810–3.
33. Trief D, Marquezan MC, Rapuano CJ, Prescott CR. Pediatric corneal transplants. Curr Opin Ophthalmol. 2017;28(5):477–84.

Index

© The Editor(s) (if applicable) and The Author(s), under exclusive license to
Springer Nature Switzerland AG 2023
A. Traish, V. P. Douglas (eds.), *Pediatric Ocular Surface Disease*,
https://doi.org/10.1007/978-3-031-30562-7

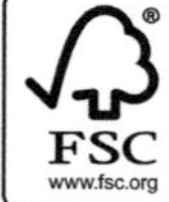

If you have any concerns about our products,
you can contact us on
ProductSafety@springernature.com

In case Publisher is established outside the EU,
the EU authorized representative is:
Springer Nature Customer Service Center GmbH
Europaplatz 3, 69115 Heidelberg, Germany

Printed by Libri Plureos GmbH
in Hamburg, Germany